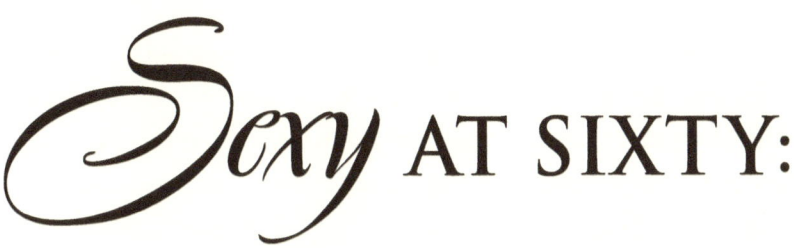 AT SIXTY:

Live Well & Happy
Men & Women over Fifty!

BY PEGGY L. HEADLUND

Strategic Book Group
Durham, Connecticut

Strategic Book Group
P.O. Box 333
Durham CT 06422
www.StrategicBookClub.com

ISBN 978-1-60976-865-2

Printed in the United States of America

Book Design: Linda W. Rigsbee

Dedication

I dedicate this book to my family, friends, and classmates living in the second half of their lives. You have faced a myriad of challenges, you've struggled for health and happiness along the way, but now it's time to live well and prosper.

Acknowledgments

Cover Photos – Marco Meza, a wonderful photographer from Playa del Carmen, Quintana Roo, Mexico took the pictures on the covers just before my sixtieth birthday. He specializes in composition photos with no touch-ups, completely natural. For me, it was a revelation, and definitely helped to lift my sagging self-esteem, because the only makeup I'm wearing is lip-gloss.

Photo at Back of Book – Thank you to my nephew, Lukas VanDyke, for his fine art photography as seen in the picture of the author at the back of this book. Thank you for always being so cheerful and professional. You are a delightful person. Everyone should be as lucky as I am to have you for a nephew and photographer.

Advice – I extend a huge, warm, and loving thank you to my husband, Donald. Thank you for listening patiently to all my ideas, and for giving me advice about the direction or tone of a subject. Thank you for taking us out to eat if I'm working towards a deadline, or if I am high on a writing frenzy. Thank you for supporting me both in my fiction and non-fiction ministry and my music ministry, and for praying with me about the direction of the ministries. Donald, sweet man, your love is precious to me. I'll never be able to thank you enough in this lifetime.

Inspiration – Most of all I'd like to thank Jesus Christ, my Savior, for his forgiveness, grace, guidance, and inspiration. Thank you, dear Shepherd, the gift belongs to you, my Maker. I pray that I will always use it wisely to glorify and honor you.

Foreword

We have all struggled with aging issues over the years. Peggy, unlike many of us, actually decided to do something about it, and she never gives up. She is a student of physical fitness and mobility, cellular metabolism, molecular genetics, cardiology, cell structure and function, human anatomy and physiology, women's and men's health issues, nutrition, nutritional healing and supplements, and naturopathy. She has diligently searched for the answers to a number of problems caused by age and the changes we experience in our bodies, and she has encouraged me to help her. If one purported solution didn't work, then she continued to seek an alternative answer to alleviate the condition.

She has attended classes at UCLA, read and collected innumerable books on the topics, followed on-line and doctor-supported research, and done her homework. She has consulted many doctors, and kept an open mind about methods used to resolve problems. Together we have searched for the answers of how to have continued health through the aging process. Sometimes we stumbled onto a solution by accident. Other times the solutions offered didn't work or relieve the pain. The whole process has taken decades to figure out, but finally we have arrived at a comfortable place where we've learned to manage the maladies.

I encouraged Peggy to write this book because she has accumulated a wealth of information over the last thirty years. People ask her questions about health and beauty everywhere we go, even on vacation. We discovered the information that she presents to you in our learning curve.

Writing a non-fiction book took Peggy away from her first love, fiction. I had to smile because she couldn't complete the book without writing an anecdote for you at the beginning of each chapter to illustrate the surprising things that happen in life. I enjoyed the humor, and we hope that you will enjoy it too, and find the book helpful for *your* continued health in the future.

Donald C. Headlund

Table of Contents

Sex Appeal 1

Anecdote

The woman gazed at her man with disdain and grumped with melodramatic emphasis, *"Old, that's not something I wanted to be when I grew up!"*

The man replied evenly and quietly, as he didn't want to incite her further, "Old or dead, what other choices do you have?"

"I have plenty of choices," she quibbled, and then snapped at him, *"and you know it!"*

"I don't know what you're so worried about anyway. You're beautiful. Men still hit on you all the time," he responded as he raised his eyebrows and smiled at her handsomely.

"You just say that because you remember me when I was young, and so when you look at me, you see me through your own personal filter," she smirked at him and lifted her chin in a challenge.

"That's not true," he answered as he stared seriously right into her eyes so that he could make his point. *"You are beautiful,"* he said insistently. Besides, he wanted to get off this topic as soon as possible before she asked him a trick question, and he stuck his foot in his mouth.

"I'm glad *you* think so," She frowned at him, harrumphed, and didn't believe that they had resolved anything.

He turned back to his newspaper, and said under his breath, "Phew! I'm glad we're finished with that topic. Sex appeal is a touchy subject."

What Is Sex Appeal?

Sexy to Your Spouse – A wise person once said that if you maintain your sex appeal to the opposite sex, you would ensure that you're still sexy to your spouse. It's difficult to feel appealing when a person isn't on top of their game physically, emotionally, mentally, and spiritually. These complex bodies dispensed to us by our Maker hold secrets, which we don't always understand.

A Learned Desire – Sex appeal is something we learn at a very young age. It is everywhere we look, any place we buy, and in almost all the materials we read, except for scientific journals, and it could show up there too. A male classmate at my twentieth high school reunion remarked, "*Everyone* feels awkward when they're in high school." That is because young people actively seek their individual brand of sex appeal, something that sets them apart from the crowd.

Different for Everyone – Sex appeal is anything that will attract the opposite sex to you. It can be a person's physique, coloring, hair, voice, smell, intelligence, hobbies, sense of humor, spirituality, clothing, degree of femininity or masculinity, or a combination of these factors. It's probably different for everyone. Tall and outrageously attractive men draw my attention, but that attraction hasn't always served me the best. What we found sexy when we were young changes, as we grow older.

What Makes a Person Sexy in Their Second Half?

Variations – Successful men attract a certain group of women.

Men who have reduced their lives to a backpack, and have the courage to pursue the things that they love attract another group of women. Some people dislike people who don't have an opinion, or in other words, they like people who speak their minds. Other folks don't like such people, not if the subject is offensive or inappropriate. Intelligence might be the sexiest characteristic that appeals to the person.

Different Goals – When we were younger, many of us were nesters. We had a desire to build a home and relationship that had security, the latter being an important factor. In the second half, financial security might not matter as much if the person has already earned it.

Fishing for Attraction

Role Model – The woman was on vacation. She invariably ran into men who approached her in the gym, at the cabana, in the water, in a restaurant, strolling down the sidewalk, or at the bar, and desired to have a conversation with her. The woman learned much about the type of man who was attracted to her, and many of them happened to be eight to fifteen years younger.

One man said to the woman, "Of course I'm older than you."

She asked how old he was, and he told her that he was fifty-two. She was eight years his senior, and contemplated telling him that she was younger. However, she felt that it was important to respond with the truth, because she didn't want to mislead anyone.

Opening Up – What the men didn't know was whether the woman was attracted to them or not. Sometimes she was, and other times she was not. The woman didn't mind talking to the men if they opened up about their lives. She found that interesting. On her last trip to Hawaii, she met three men, two of whom desired to have the same profession as she had. She took pleasure in encouraging them. One man followed her around everywhere she went, even to the women's room, just so he could ask more questions. The woman began to question his sincerity!

Embrace Each Birthday with Delight

Sexy Sweat – For the wife's sixtieth birthday, her husband took her to the big island of Hawaii. It was the best birthday that she had ever experienced. The day began in the gym on the bicycle. She sat on a recumbent bicycle in the middle of a row of middle-aged men in their forties and fifties. They teased her incessantly and marveled at her level of endurance on the hill program.

The wife remarked, "It's probably because I have a bicycle at home."

She rode the bike for an hour on the hill program, and traveled an imaginary twenty-four miles. She dusted all the men around her. Covered with sweat and with no makeup, her presence there in the fitness center appealed to the men. That fact dumbfounded her, and she wondered why. She figured that sex appeal was a nebulous trait.

Hope for the Future – When she finished her program, one man stopped her, and commented, "I've been on this bicycle for ninety minutes, and I haven't even reached twenty miles yet." The wife pondered how to answer his comment, and felt that the truth would give him hope for the future.

She replied, "Well thanks, and today is my sixtieth birthday!" She smirked at him, and he rolled his eyes at her and laughed jovially.

Attraction – Later that day, while she and her husband reclined in their cabana, the same man stopped by their cabana, and cheerily said, "Happy Birthday!"

The wife suspected that there was a conversation about her age over on his side of the pool because soon thereafter, several more men stopped by to wish her a happy birthday. The wife worried that her husband might feel jealous, but he didn't. He liked the fact that other men still found his wife attractive. Throughout the afternoon, a steady stream of people found a reason to come over and talk with the wife, both men and women.

An Interest in Others' Lives – When the wife went to the beach, she didn't read a book, she wrote a book, because that is where she felt the most inspired. The fact that she was a writer often drew inquisitive folks. They asked questions about her appearance, physical fitness, beauty secrets, her work, and the types of books that she wrote. It gave her an opportunity to hand a business card to each of them, and accept a business card in return, which brought even more people to their cabana. Once the guests noticed that she was approachable, the crowd didn't hold back. The wife talked to people from all over the world, and they expressed some amazing things about themselves. She found interesting and exciting story lines by learning about their lives.

Her husband teased her and said, "Lilia makes friends, wherever she goes!" Lilia was the main character in the wife's fictional books, and indeed the wife did make friends, wherever she went!

Age Differences Don't Deter Attraction

Older men were always attracted to the wife, and nothing had changed in that quarter. It was probably the reason that she was married to a magnificent specimen of a man, and was with him for thirty years. His appearance was dark in coloring, with handsome olive skin, and a physique that he diligently maintained. He appeared to be around sixty years of age, when, in fact, he was seventy-seven years old. He was extremely smart, kind, loving, and often knew what was best for her before she did. *Now, that's sexy,* the wife thought.

The Desire for Sex Appeal Doesn't Disappear with Age

Almost everyone wants to believe that he or she still has sex appeal, especially as we grow older. It's a difficult characteristic to set aside when we've worked at maintaining it most of our lives. No one wants to feel unloved. It doesn't matter how old you are.

Health Problems Derail Sex Appeal

It was difficult for me to feel attractive and physically fit with arthritis, sciatica, numerous leg injuries, a shrinking spine, neck pain, and a slouching posture. Depression and hormonal imbalances caused me to struggle for a regulated state of mental health. I wrestled for emotional stability and the expression of love with a longtime partner in marriage, who had his own issues to conquer. I scrutinized the future of my changing career goals, and questioned my spirituality, which I thought was solidly secure in terms of my relationship with God.

How do people ever get to a point where they feel happy with the way they look, feel, act, and exist? Finding the answers to all these hurdles has taken many years, but Don, and I have finally arrived at the point where we can exist in our second half with wellness and happiness. Because I feel better physically, emotionally, mentally, and spiritually, *now I feel sexy too!*

Weight Control

Anecdote

The man remarked to the woman, "Well, if you're *so* unhappy with your weight, why don't you go consult a nutritionist?"

The woman retorted, *"You think I'm fat!"*

"No, I didn't say that. There are many people where I work who have visited a certain nutritionist, and are very happy with the results. Why don't you give it a try?" He suggested persuasively, since he knew that she was obsessed with her weight.

She grimaced while he continued to peer at her, and then deplored, "Oh all right, *I'll go!*" She went to the nutritionist, and successfully lost the weight that annoyed her.

Six months later, they drove in the car to their ski condominium. She said quietly to the man, "You need to lose a little weight honey." He glared at her with anger, snapped his mouth shut, and they drove in silence for the next few hours because he didn't think he was fat.

The woman asserted in his silence, "Well, when we get really old we won't have to worry about it because we'll be skinny."

He looked at her curiously, and finally broke the silence, "Why will we be skinny?"

"We'll be skinny because we won't be able to open any of the super-sealed food containers!" She said and laughed. He smiled at her, and chuckled.

A Tale of Roller Coaster Weight

Family-Perpetuated Stigmas – If you asked the wife how much she weighed on any given day of her life, she'd probably be able to tell you. If it wasn't enough to be a healthy-looking farm girl in the time and influence of Twiggy, she had her mother to point it out to her regularly. Her grandmother was obsessed with her weight and appearance, too, and never weighed more than ninety pounds, even though she was tall for her age. Her grandmother passed on her obsession to the wife's mother, who was always a petite and skinny woman. The mother passed that obsession on to the wife.

When the wife was but ten years old, her mom took her aside for a heart-to-heart talk about her weight. The young woman had already reached her full height of five-feet, six inches, and indeed for a short time, was the tallest girl in her class. She wasn't a fat child, but she wasn't skinny either. A description of wholesome and sturdy rang true. Her mom explained to her that it wasn't normal to have a lump of flesh above her knee. Maybe it wasn't right for the mother with her scrawny frame, but it *was* normal for the daughter. That lump that her mother spurned was muscle resulting from heavy farm chores of lifting and throwing bales of hay and straw, toting milk pails weighing fifty pounds or more in each arm, lifting feed sacks, and training and working with cattle and horses. Aerobic exercise didn't fit into the daily mix of their activities, unless they played 4-H softball. Many years later, the wife learned about the value of cardiovascular exercise.

Continuous Struggle to Control Weight – It turns out that the mother was right about one thing: The wife had a weight problem all of her life. She tried just about everything in the cycle of things. As a young woman and dairy princess in Minnesota, she lost the extra pounds by eating egg whites, cornflakes, and oranges. That was definitely boring, but she was motivated! Later, she tried all the weight management organizations available to her at the time. She lost the weight, and then her boss pronounced that she was too skinny! Diet after diet came into her life and helped her to manage the weight for brief periods.

Injuries and Middle Age – When the wife entered her fifties, she was around ten pounds overweight, but extremely physically fit. She ran eight to ten miles a day. In the process, she experienced seven leg injuries, and couldn't walk normally for two years. She felt so jealous of other people who could place one foot in front of another without a problem, since she spent a great portion of that time on crutches and in a wheelchair. In fact, she took a trip to Hawaii with her petite mom, and they shared the wheelchair!

Help from a Nutritionist – All that time without proper aerobic exercise caused the wife to gain fifteen more pounds, and then she had twenty-five pounds to lose. The wife's frustration reached a peak level, and so her husband stepped in and suggested that she should consult a popular nutritionist. At the time, she was highly insulted, but her husband encouraged her, and so she went.

Starvation Mode – The first thing the nutritionist taught the wife was that she wasn't eating enough. The nutritionist and the wife catalogued everything she had eaten the two days before her consultation, and it didn't amount to more than six hundred calories a day. He explained to her that she had completely and successfully shut down her metabolism, and propelled her body into a starvation mode. Her body stopped burning calories effectively, and the result was that she had a body fat content over thirty percent. She was now officially obese! *Fat* is also something she never wanted to be when she grew up!

Type of Metabolism – The nutritionist poked her finger, and took a little blood to find out what type of metabolism the wife had, and then he would know what food to recommend to her. It turned out that she had the metabolism of an athlete. Only three percent of the people in the world had this type of metabolism. The wife guessed that was good news because an athlete burned the categories of carbohydrates, protein, and fat equally. The catch was the carbohydrates. They experimented with bread the first week, rice the second week, pasta the third week, and tortillas the fourth week with no significant weight loss for the wife. They finally tried potatoes, and that was it! Potatoes were the carbohydrate that she burned. Thank goodness that it was potatoes, because she loved them!

Five Meals a Day to the Perfect Size – The nutritionist gave her around twelve to fifteen-hundred calories to eat a day. She attested that she always ate more than that, but she still lost weight. He spread the food out into three big meals and two little meals. The wife was amazed that she could eat so much and lose weight. The nutritionist also taught her how to achieve quick weight loss with a short-term plan of fish and vegetables. The wife was a happy woman! She consulted with the nutritionist every week for a year, and then a family crisis kept her from returning. She continued to follow his plan, though. Her weight stabilized, and she stopped losing weight. Size 4 fitted her perfectly.

Too Thin and Wrinkled – As the wife approached her mid-fifties, she became involved in show business again, and did a couple big shows. Six hours of dancing a day caused her to lose another twelve pounds, and she became downright skinny. If you looked at her face back then, the skin sagged so badly that she declared to her husband that she looked just like a very well known mature *male* actor with bright blue eyes. She hated how her face looked, but was pleased that a Size 2 was slightly big on her, since she believed the old adage that a woman could never be too rich or too thin. The husband told the wife that she looked like a scarecrow, and that it wasn't attractive, and so the wife allowed herself to gain a few pounds to fill in the wrinkles.

Poor Elimination – Now, the wife arrived at her late fifties. She hadn't eaten red meat for thirty years. She hadn't eaten bread, rice, or pasta for eight years. Her whole system became so sluggish that she only had proper elimination twice a week. She felt miserable, crabby, and undesirable. She added bread back into her diet, and immediately gained five pounds, which made her angry. It seemed that she needed fiber more than she needed bread.

Subscribe to Fiber and Lose the Weight for Good

Amount Needed – The National Cancer Institute and the American Diabetes Association recommend 20-35 grams of fiber a day. You can lose up to ten unwanted pounds in a year simply by eating fiber. Print out a list from the web of foods with high fiber, and start eating more fiber today. You might be surprised at the number of foods you like, which have more fiber.

Fiber for Every Meal – Revamp your eating plan. Spread your fiber out through the day, until your body becomes accustomed to it. Adding fiber to your nutritional plan doesn't mean that you can add unlimited fats. The fiber will drag the fat out of your system, but it won't straighten out an imbalance in food input and activity output. Put yourself on the eighty/twenty plan. Eat sensibly eighty percent of the time, and eat whatever you want twenty percent of the time, but keep the fiber in your diet all the time.

Between Meals Fiber – If you become hungry in between meals, eat raw and unsalted almonds. There is 1 gram of fiber in one table-spoon of almonds. The truth is that you probably won't become hungry between meals because the fiber provides a sense of fullness all the time.

Fiber Every Day – One thing the wife knew was that when she didn't eat the fiber each day, it only took one day for her to bloat-up like a cow after eating beet pulp! When the wife and the husband returned from Hawaii, her clothes felt a little tight on her. That's because they took all her fruits and vegetables away from her in the agricultural inspection, and she didn't have any fiber for a day.

Solution for Feelings of Deprivation – The wife thought that she was getting too old to deprive herself anymore. Thirty years without beef seemed a little extreme, but it was good advice given to her by a famous doctor after she had endometrial cancer. Not eating bread for eight years almost stretched her discipline as much as a rubber band bursting. A delightful slice of cracked wheat bread once a day satisfied her completely. If you're tired of deprivation, throw out your scale, and simply wait out the weight. Eat your daily fiber, and watch the pounds disappear naturally.

Irvingia for Weight Loss, High Cholesterol, and Blood Glucose Levels

Irvingia is a derivative developed from the dika nuts of wild mango, African mango, or bush mango trees. This high-fiber nut is composed of fourteen percent fiber, which might be the reason that it works for weight loss, lowering bad cholesterol, raising good cholesterol, and lowering blood glucose levels. Test groups lost weight and lowered their body fat significantly. Irvingia is new to the health food industry, and therefore, research and studies continue.

Eat Proteins for Metabolism

Proteins are important to get your metabolism moving, but stay within the suggested range of four to six ounces of protein for lunch and supper. If you don't gain weight, then add a few more ounces. You'll burn more protein with more exercise.

Avoid Foods with Toxins

Coal Tar – Don't eat processed foods if you can avoid them. If a food or a drink has an artificial color, flavor, or scent, chances are that it has coal tar in it, which is a carcinogenic. Carcinogens cause cancer.

Nitrates – Packaged deli meats often contain nitrates, which also cause cancer. There are some packaged deli meats, which don't contain nitrates, such as Black Forest Ham or Turkey. Get into the habit of reading the labels.

Diethylstilbestrol (DES) – Buy organic foods whenever possible. The beef and poultry industries used a hormone called diethylstilbestrol (DES) in the 1960s. DES causes breast cancer, and cancer of the reproductive organs. Supposedly, the beef and poultry industries discontinued the use of DES by the 1970s. Many people disagree, and claim that its use is still prevalent in the meat sold in the United States today.

Pesticides – Pesticides used in foods that are not organic pose another potential problem. When we eat pesticides, we accept the risks that go with the territory: birth defects, miscarriage, and damage to the nerves, Parkinson's disease, and certain types of cancer.

Focus on Energy and Health

If you are a member of the human race, at some point you will have a desire to eat something that isn't good for you. When the temptation hits you, remember that eating the right food fuels you with energy and health, and don't go crazy.

Exercise and Injuries 3

Anecdote

On a very steep ski slope on the backside of the mountain, the man cried out in pain, *"Ouch! Something popped in my knee!"*

"The woman asked with concern, "Do you think that you can ski down?"

"I think so, if you ski over to the other side of the mountain and get me an Ace bandage for my knee," he said with confidence and a little too much bravado. She gazed at him doubtfully, and then shot off down the hill.

She whisked up to the ski patrol at the bottom of the slope and announced, "My husband's standing to the side of the ski slope up there. He's hurt. Could you go up and get him?"

"What color is his jacket?" The ski patrol asked perfunctorily.

"It's white, purple, and black," she replied with a grimace. She knew the husband wouldn't appreciate her decision.

The ski patrol pulled the sled to the front of the lift line, hopped on the chairlift with the sled, and went up to find the man. The woman waited in line, and then followed the ski patrol to the top of the mountain.

When the ski patrol found the man, he asked, "Are you hurt?"

The man replied with surprise, "No, I'm fine. I'm waiting for my wife to bring me an Ace bandage. I don't need to go down in the sled."

Shortly after, the woman arrived on the scene, and the ski patrol tersely said to her, "*He* says he's *not* hurt."

The man peered at the woman with anger, and she defended herself, "Don't blame me. I did what any good woman would do. I brought help. *Now get in the sled!*"

He frowned at her. She pressed her lips together in a thin line, which meant that she wasn't buying his story. The man reluctantly sat down in the sled and swung his legs inside. The ski patrol strapped him in, and skied briskly and evenly with him to the bottom, where they hooked the man in the sled to a snowmobile to haul him up over the mountain to the other side.

The ski patrol told the woman, "Come and get him in at the first aid station at the Main Lodge."

"Okay," she replied, and scurried off towards the chairlift.

She schussed as fast and wide as she could down four runs before she arrived back at Canyon Lodge. She hurriedly stowed her gear, and jogged up the short hill to the car. She hopped in and drove seven miles to the Main Lodge to pick up the man. She discovered her husband laying on a cot in the first air station where the ski patrol had strapped on a brace.

"I can't remove the brace," announced the ski patrol, "because of the liability. Either you or your husband will have to remove it if he doesn't go to the hospital."

The man scowled at the woman again for good measure, and said irritably, "*I'm fine.*"

He removed the brace, stood up, and hobbled after the woman to the car. The woman drove him back to their place, where the man applied an ice pack directly onto the skin of his injured knee. He tied the ice on with a dishtowel. It was the woman's birthday, and the man had just put the kibosh on the celebratory trip.

He said consolingly, "Don't worry honey, I'll be all right to ski tomorrow."

She wasn't certain about that, but decided not to buck him on it, and so they sat down and played Scrabble for four hours, and then removed the ice and went to bed. The next morning the man awoke and peered at his knee with horror where three giant balloons of skin filled with fluid hung from his kneecap. The ice applied directly to his skin the night before had frost bitten his skin.

He showed the woman the gagging mess, which was his leg, and said with determination, "If I put a bandage on it, I can probably ski on it."

"*You're an idiot!*" retorted the woman, and she bundled him into the car and drove him to the local ski surgeon's office.

The ski surgeon came out into the waiting room, and peeped at the chairs filled with a crop of new injuries. He looked around, and then smiled and turned to the man, "You're next!" He turned to the woman and ordered, "Come with me." She followed her husband and the surgeon into the examining room. The ski surgeon took a quick look, and inquired of the woman, "Did he have any breakfast?"

"No, I brought him here instead," the woman replied with concern.

"Good, we'll operate in two hours before the ligament has a chance to shrink up," the surgeon replied cheerily.

The man gazed at his wife in shock, and said, "It didn't feel like it was anything serious."

She knowingly shook her head back and forth at the man, and sneered, "*Right!*"

Athletes Eventually Incur Injuries: The Wife's Story

Excessive Strain – The wife was born with a Type A Personality. She realized that sometimes it was a good thing, and other times it was not. She entered her fifties as a running fool. She purchased a fancy treadmill. It could do everything. She could run uphill, downhill, and train in a number of programs. She sped along on her machine at six miles per hour. She took special pride in being able to run so fast and well because back in high school, when the school administered the physical fitness tests, she couldn't even run a half-mile. The wife and the husband also had a stationary bicycle, which she discontinued using when they purchased the treadmill. The wife's routine consisted of two, four-mile to five-mile running sessions a day, and additional exercises to strengthen the upper body.

Plantar Fasciitis and a Sprained Ankle – Just before the husband and the wife departed for a business conference in Arizona, the arch fell on her right foot, and the doctor pronounced that she had plantar fasciitis. It didn't deter the wife because she could tolerate the pain. She'd always had a high threshold for pain. With orthotics in her shoes, she continued to run, even after the arch fell on her left foot too. At the conference, she ran around the resort property, tripped in a pothole, and sprained her ankle. That slowed her down a little. She wrapped it up, iced it, and hobbled around for the remainder of the conference.

Torn Ligament – Once back at home, the husband and the wife repacked their suitcases, and departed for Mammoth Mountain in the High Sierra Nevada Mountains where they had a condominium right next to Canyon Lodge. They popped on their skis and headed for the 11,015-foot cornice. She leaped off the cornice with all the confidence of an experienced and advanced skier. On the first extremely steep schuss, she felt something tear in her left knee. She felt certain that it was her anterior cruciate ligament. She didn't hear it pop, so she believed that it was only a small rip. You can probably guess what happened next. She bandaged it up, slipped on a brace, and returned to the mountain to ski, and you think that the man in the anecdote was an idiot!

Truncated Posterior and Medial Meniscus – Back at home again, she limped around and nursed her injuries, when her left hip, which was always loose, slid out of place slightly. One morning, when she walked their two beautiful little Westies, they bounded forward at another dog, and the medial meniscus in her left knee truncated both in the front and the back. She fell into the street, and shrieked loud enough to bring people out of their houses. Two helpful pool men carried her home as she blubbered with tears, and the dogs barked wildly at the commotion.

Knees and Vulnerability – The doctor explained to her that knees carried the body's weight and endured a number of factors that have to do with stability. She asked the doctor if her knees acted like the suspension and stability system in her truck.

He told her, "Yes, they keep everything balanced. The knee can absorb a vertical force when you jump off something up to seven times your body's weight, but they are vulnerable to horizontal or rotational movements."

Crutches, a Wheelchair, and Surgery – That was the end of exercise for the wife. She was completely undone and knocked off her fitness routine, and came to depend on crutches and a wheelchair for a period spanning two years. Months of doctor visits ensued, until she finally found a surgeon who professed that he could fix it. Of course, she had the surgery. She couldn't wait to be able to walk again, and felt highly concerned about what the lack of exercise would do to her.

Perpetuation of Injuries – The husband chastised the wife, "You got exactly what you deserved when you didn't allow any of the injuries to heal properly."

She realized that it was like the electricity going off room by room in the house, until the whole house lied quiet and dysfunctional. A limp with one leg imbalanced the spine, and perpetuated other injuries when the body didn't move with fluidity.

The Value of Exercise

Longevity – Exercise is a valuable tool in reducing the risks of obesity, diabetes, cardiovascular disease, and some types of cancers. The exercise doesn't have to be excessive, thirty minutes of moderate-intensity exercise five or more days a week lowers the risks considerably. Exercise promotes a healthy sleep pattern. The simple fact is that if you exercise consistently, *you will live longer*. Regular exercise helps to burn calories, and improves lung function. Choose an exercise routine with strength training, aerobic exercise, and balance and flexibility.

Strength and Endurance for Activities – Make a commitment to your exercise routine and reap the benefits. Stronger bones and muscles, along with endurance, maintain a fit body, which can enjoy golf, skiing, and tons of other activities.

Shape – It also gives you shape. Shape ensures that you still have sex appeal, and it improves self-esteem.

Endorphins – There are enough pressures and anxieties endured, as we grow older, why not utilize the wonderful mood lifter and natural pain reliever you achieve through the influx of endorphins from exercise? It helps in the control of depression.

Blood Pressure and Cholesterol – Exercise helps to lower your blood pressure and cholesterol.

Mental Acuity – Exercise improves your mental acuity. If you're pondering something, and can't figure it out, get up and move!

Other Advantages – Exercise boosts your immune system, as well as the metabolism of glucosamine, which helps your joints. Exercise reduces our sensitivity to insulin.

Commitment – It doesn't matter at what level you start, but do make a commitment to at least three hours a week, and get connected with the youthful you.

Elongated Muscles – The lump above the wife's knee, which annoyed her mom when she was young, disappeared with cardio-vascular exercise. Aerobic exercise lengthened the muscles to a smooth elongated appearance.

You're Never Too Old to Start Exercising

Shaped Shoes – Many people buy into the theory that when you stop an activity, it's over. That is not true, and the wife proved it. Two years without exercise other than gardening and house chores left her in poor physical condition. The doctor told her not to run anymore, but to choose a different cardiovascular exercise. Long before the public knew about shaped shoes, she had cut an ad out of a model's magazine for the fantastic Swiss-engineered shoes. They were a model's best kept secret. The constant balancing in the shoes exercised the muscles, both in the front and the back, all the way from a person's ankles up to the chest and neck.

End Chiropractor Visits – After the debacle with the leg injuries, the wife had to visit the chiropractor three times a week to push her left hip and her neck back into place. The time to go there cut a huge portion of available work time out of her schedule, and frustrated her to the point of temper. When she began to walk in the shoes, she could feel her spine straightening out, and her chest thrust forward. Her hips, knees, and ankles snapped and crackled, until everything was back in alignment, and then she didn't have to visit the chiropractor anymore.

An Overall Conditioned Physique – She walked four miles, or one hour, in the shoes every day, and continued the routine with a half hour of upper body exercises, and a series of stretches. It only took a couple of months for her to achieve a conditioned physique. She especially liked the fact that it made her abdominal muscles and back muscles strong enough to stand up straight. The amazing shaped shoes did their job. They also caused a lawyer to discharge her from a jury in a trial where the woman had been rear-ended, and now had to go to the chiropractor every day for pain relief. The woman laughed with joy when she understood that the "special shoes" could do almost anything except order opera tickets, and wash the dishes!

Sciatica

Causes – When the wife began working at her desk every day, she developed a severe case of sciatica. It was even more painful than the plantar fasciitis! The wife did her research. She discovered that there were many different causes for sciatica: deterioration in the disks of the back, which is related to aging; lifting or twisting the back regularly; driving in a vehicle for prolonged periods of time; sitting at a desk all day; and diabetes, which can increase the risk of nerve damage. The husband and the wife surmised about what had caused it, and couldn't decide on any single factor, other than the amount of time that she spent at the computer each day.

Painful Effects – The wife hated the excruciating pain. It shot through her like an electric shock wave from her spinal cord, through the buttock and hip area, and straight down the back of her legs. She commented to her husband that it felt like someone poked her legs with pins and needles. Although, it affected most people on one side more than the other, for the wife the pain was equally debilitating on both sides. The pain was so agonizing that she had to take super-strength aspirin every four hours to tolerate it, and then had to sleep on a heating pad at night to attain any sleep at all. Once the heating pad clicked off, the wife woke up and the pain started all over again.

Contraindications of Cortisone Injection – A girlfriend explained to the wife that her husband's sciatica disappeared after a shot of cortisone. The husband and wife lived by one simple rule: Don't put anything unnatural into the body, unless there is no other solution. The wife searched the contraindications of cortisone in her extensive library. The results were shocking to her. She discovered that the contraindications for the drug were worse than the illness. There were multiple contraindications in each category, thirty-seven in all. They ranged from fluid retention, osteoporosis, abdominal distention to facial distortion, convulsions, latent diabetes, glaucoma, and many more. The findings ended any desire to obtain a cortisone injection.

A Symptom, Not a Disorder – The first thing the wife learned was that sciatica was not a disorder. Sciatica was a symptom from something else that had gone awry. There were a number of disorders: a narrowing in one or more areas of the spine; a vertebra, which drifted forward over another vertebra, and the bone pinched the sciatic nerve; spinal tumors; trauma from an accident; damaged sciatic nerve. The wife's was none of those. It was Piriformis Syndrome. The wife ascertained that the piriformis muscle began at the lower spine, and connected to the thighbone. When the muscle became tight, it pressured her sciatic nerve and caused spasms of pain to shoot down her legs.

Stop What You're Doing – There are a number of ways to approach the problem from physical therapy to an injection of corticosteroid, and from prescription drugs to surgery. The wife chose physical therapy. She searched online for a manual that would explain how to do the physical therapy, and found a good one. The manual told her that the first thing she had to do was stop exercising. The wife didn't want to hear that! She wondered if the shaped shoes had aggravated it, and so stopped using them for a while. She returned to the recumbent bicycle for exercise and rode twenty-two miles on the hill program every day, but Sunday. She found that the bicycle didn't aggravate the sciatica, and continued with that tact for a while.

Other Helpful Remedies – The wife tried a few other remedies too. She placed gel insoles in her shoes to support her feet better.

The husband hung an exercise bar on the eaves at the back of their house. The wife retrieved a stool to reach the bar, and then stepped off the stool and hung from the bar as long as her hands could stand it. That gave her immediate relief. She could feel and hear the vertebra decompress and extend with the weight of her body pulling downward. From that point on, she diligently took the time to hang from the bar several times a day. She even had positive thoughts about recovering the half-inch of height that she'd lost since high school!

Walking in the Swimming Pool – The other thing that helped the wife immensely was walking around in the swimming pool. The pressure from the water was equal all around her body, and so the water forced anything that was out of balance to correct itself. The wife set aside time to walk around in the swimming pool each day. The pain retreated, and only returned when she sat back down at her desk.

Improved Posture at the Computer – The wife noticed that she slouched while she worked on her computer. She bought a drafter's chair, leaned forward, and hooked her feet on the metal bar, which helped tremendously. To ensure an ongoing corrected posture, she bought a shoulder brace, which pulled her shoulders back and forced her to sit up properly. She wore it over her clothes, whenever she worked at her desk.

Self-Evaluation and Stretches – The manual for sciatica came with a self-evaluation procedure and a number of stretches. Soon the wife discovered the stretches that helped her the most, and she did them every day.

Bend the Knees – The wife discerned by accident that if she bent her knees when she bent over, it helped to stretch the piriformis muscle. She began a new routine. When she dried her hair, she bent her knees, and dried her hair upside down. By the time that her almost waist-length hair was dry, the muscle had stretched out.

Disappearance of Sciatica – The wife's sciatica completely disappeared using the techniques outlined above, and she finally experienced relief.

Commitment to an Exercise Routine

Currently, the wife's daily exercise routine includes the following: one hour of gardening; twenty-two miles on the uphill program on the recumbent bicycle with fifteen minutes of neck stretches at the end of the ride; thirty push-ups; resistance sit-ups; hip stretches; hanging on the bar in the backyard; and occasionally walking in the swimming pool. The wife wears the shaped shoes around the house.

Stretches for Neck Pain

Sensitivity of Carotid Arteries – The carotid arteries in the neck are sensitive to sudden movements or popping of the neck. When you do the stretches outlined below, make your movements slow and easy, and count to thirty for each stretch. Don't place an undue strain on the neck.

Number of Sets – Work through all the stretches in the order prescribed, and then start over again. Perform five sets of all the stretches.

Chin to Shoulder Stretch – Turn your head and set your chin as close to your relaxed right shoulder as you can, and count to thirty. Then reverse your chin and repeat the same stretch over the left shoulder, and count to thirty.

Head Over Shoulder Stretch – Hang your head back over your right shoulder, and count to thirty. Then hang your head back over your left shoulder, and count to thirty.

Head Towards Shoulder Stretch – Hold your head with your right hand, pull it to the side towards your right shoulder, and count to thirty. Don't drop your chin. Position your head so that it is as close to parallel with the shoulder as is comfortable. Then hold the head with your left hand, pull it to the side towards your left shoulder, and count to thirty.

Chin Down and Back Stretch – Lower your chin to your chest, and count to thirty. Then hang it straight back, and count to thirty.

Disappearance of Neck Pain – Consistent stretching of the neck alleviates chronic neck pain caused from repeated motion or static positions. The stretches alleviated the wife's neck pain that she had from sitting at her desk for hours each day.

Shapely Biceps and Triceps

A Device for Motion Fluidity – The wife had an interesting device for push-ups. They were handles that swiveled, so that her biceps *and* triceps received a workout with each push-up.

In the up position of the push-up, the wife gripped the handles straight up and down. As she lowered herself to the bottom of the push-up, she gradually swiveled the handles to a horizontal position, which caused her elbows to stick out to the side. When she returned to the up position, she swiveled the handles back to the straight up and down position.

Shapely Arms – A neighbor commented on the shapeliness of the wife's upper arms for her age, and she explained that the swivel handles were the reason why.

Strong Stomach Muscles Support Your Back

Belly Button Press – Any exercise, in which the stomach muscle presses the belly button down, as if it pressed it into the spine, is effective for creating rock hard stomach muscles.

Sit-Up and Press Down – 1) Lie on the floor with bent legs, and feet resting flat on the floor. 2) Sit up halfway, and extend the arms straight out in front of you on either side of your bent legs. 3) Use the stomach muscles to press your belly button down, as if you pressed it into your spine, with as much effort as possible. 4) While in that position, alternately lift your legs off the floor to a slow and deliberate count of twenty-five.

Perform fifteen of the twenty-five count sit-ups. Try to do at least five at a time before resting. Eventually, you'll be able to do all fifteen without a break.

Keep a Shapely Little Round Belly – The wife attempted to rid herself of the detested little round belly, which she'd had all her life. Every woman in her family, including cousins, had it too. Her sister, who was quite slender, still had the little round belly. The wife visited a plastic surgeon and asked him for liposuction to rid her of the curse.

He asked her with a smirk, "Would you rather have a shapely little round belly, or a big ugly flap of empty skin hanging down?"

The wife cackled with laughter, and decided quickly!

Hip Stretches

Tight and Lopsided Hips – As we grow older, the hips act differently on each side for a variety of reasons. One hip might drift forward, while the other hip remains where it should. One hip might lose mobility due to an injury or imperfect position.

Hip Stretches – A posture specialist analyzed the wife's lopsided hips caused by her multiple leg injuries, and gave her a series of hip stretches to do each day to open them up, and move them back into a proper position.

Butt to the Wall Stretch – 1) Lie down perpendicular to a wall with your butt as close to the wall as you can get it. 2) Extend your legs straight up on the wall. 3) Slide your legs outward, as far apart as you can get them. Allow the weight of your legs to pull your legs even further outward.

Hold the position for around five minutes, while breathing evenly and deeply. Try to open the legs a little further each day.

Floor Bent Leg Stretch – 1) Sit down on the floor with both legs bent to the right and resting on the floor. Your weight will be on your left leg and buttock. 2) Stretch out the right leg directly behind you with extended toes. 3) Lean forward, and lie down over the left bent knee to apply more pressure. Hold the position and count to thirty.

Reverse the stretch. 1) Sit down on the floor with both legs bent to the left and resting on the floor. Your weight will be on your right leg and buttock. 2) Stretch out the left leg directly behind you with extended toes. 3) Lean forward, and lie down over the right bent knee to apply more pressure. Hold the position and count to thirty.

Hold the stretch longer if your hip doesn't move back into position.

Proper Breathing for Quality Exercise

Strength Training – Exhale the carbon dioxide from your lungs during the exertion part of the exercise. Blow it out to prevent lactic acid from building up in the muscles, which will cause stiffness and pain. You'll know when the carbon dioxide is building up because the exercise will become more difficult for you to do, and you will begin to feel fatigued and short of breath.

Exercising at Altitude – We breathe deeper and harder at altitude. Carbon dioxide will build up if you don't make a concerted effort to blow it out. The difference between a novice and an experienced skier at altitude will show up the next day when they get out of bed. The experienced skier who knows how to blow out the carbon dioxide forcefully will not feel stiff, and the novice skier will screech with pain.

The wife explained to her husband, "Friends and family have accused me of trying to kill them on the slopes, but it's not where we ski, it is how we breathe!"

Cardiovascular Exercise – Employ strong and deep breaths. Establish an inhale and exhale pattern to smooth out the strain on any hills. If you are running, inhale your breath on the first three steps, and then exhale your breath on the next two steps. This routine ensures that you inhale deeply enough to sustain you over a distance.

Flexibility Exercise – Exercises such as yoga require deep breaths from the diaphragm. Deep diaphragm breathing encourages relaxation, greater flexibility, and an ease of execution.

Sweat

Radiant Skin – A colleague from the wife's workplace arrived at the house right after the wife's workout.

She declared, "You're positively glowing!" The wife thought that the human race reserved that phrase, specifically for pregnant women, and laughed.

Flushes Toxins – What the colleague said was true, though. You might not like to sweat, but it's good for you. It flushes the toxins out of your bodies, and onto the surface of your skin. Toxins make a person age faster. Get out there and sweat, and slow down the aging process.

Wash Off Toxins – Once the toxins are lying on the surface of the skin, you'll need to remove them with a good washing. Some studies report that prolonged existence of toxins on the skin can produce dark spots on the skin.

Nerves and Pulse-Rate – Sweating has other health benefits too. We already know that it helps to cool down the body, but sweat also helps to calm nerves and regulate the pulse-rate. Whenever you become upset about something, get some brisk exercise. When you break into a sweat, you'll begin to feel better.

Exercise Clothing

Because exercise is such an everyday necessity, you'll want to get the most out of it. Wear self-wicking yoga clothing made from 85% Polyester, and 15% Elastane. The clothing wicks the sweat away from your body, and cools you during the exercise routine. When you're finished with a session, your clothes will be completely soaked, but you'll feel comfortable.

Hydration

Hydration is essential for healing, digestion, muscle use, expulsion of toxins, and almost everything else. Establish a routine, and follow it diligently.

The wife drank a bottle of water for each of the following activities: with her vitamins in the morning, while eating breakfast, while gardening, while riding the recumbent bike, for her sunning session, with her vitamins at noon, while eating lunch, while working in the afternoon, with her vitamins at dinner, and while resting during the night. That makes ten pints of water a day. Are you drinking enough water?

Longevity

Retain Mobility – Many years ago, the wife met an older man in the park, who walked his little white Bijan Frise dog every day. They discovered that they had the same date for their birthdays, only he was thirty-five years the wife's senior, an active ninety-five years old.

The man's wife had died many years before, but he continued to walk his little dog every day. He walked around the bay of the lake, down to the beach and back again. From his house, that was probably only a quarter of a mile, but he did it every day, twice a day.

The first little Bijan died, and he purchased another one, and named her the same thing as his first dog. The second Bijan died, and he purchased a third pet, and named her the same name again! He didn't walk fast, but he did walk.

The wife asked him one day how he was feeling, and he told her that he was feeling fine, and had just planted two new bushes in his yard. That is truly an amazing feat for a ninety-five-year-old man! He told her that he had developed the habit of walking every day when he retired at the age of seventy-two. The little dog and the habit of walking twice a day helped him to retain his mobility.

Loss of Mobility – Many years ago, the wife worked at a nursing home, and had volunteered in several facilities since then. The wife and the husband discussed the remarkable man who lived by the lake.

The wife said with emphasis to her husband, "Anyone who works with older folks will tell you that once they give up walking, and sit down in a wheelchair, it's all over. Most of them don't ever get back up out of the wheelchair again."

"Yeah, I know what you mean. It's like in that movie we saw, *Away from Her*. Everyone needs a role model like the man by the lake to inspire them," the husband replied with a smile.

Belly Fat

Anecdote

Summer had arrived and the woman couldn't wait to hop into her favorite shorts. She pulled them out of storage, and slipped them on. She grabbed the zipper and began to zip the pants up over her lower belly. She zipped them part way up, and they wouldn't go any further. If she tried to close the fastener, it only pushed the upper belly fat upward into a muffin top and made things worse.

"*Hoh!*" she exclaimed with frustration. "When did this happen?"

The man knew when he was treading on dangerous ground. He answered cautiously, "I suppose it happened over the winter." He shrugged his shoulders at her to indicate he really didn't know.

"Do you think I have a *big belly?*" She asked him and glared at him with anger.

"I'm not going to answer that question. It's a trick question, and I'll never get the answer right. I suppose the next thing you're going to ask me is about your butt," he said calmly with a smirk.

She snapped at him with exasperation, "*What am I going to do about this?*" She pressed her lips together in a thin line, and peevishly stared at her husband.

"I'm getting out of here while the gettin' is good!" The man said hastily and hustled out of the dressing room without another word.

The woman removed the shorts, and examined her image in the mirror. She was in postmenopause and she had just turned sixty years old. It appeared that things had shifted a bit. Her normally muscular arms and legs appeared thinner than before, and her waist was obviously bigger.

She slammed the shorts onto the floor with temper, and hollered loud enough for her husband to hear her downstairs, "*I refuse to buy a larger size!*"

She stomped on the shorts with her foot, and kicked them against the wall. The man could hear her hissy fit all the way downstairs in his office. He casually walked to the pantry, took out the calcium-magnesium-zinc bottle, extracted a pill from the bottle, and walked back upstairs with it. He handed her a glass of water and the magical little pill, which he knew would calm her down.

"Here, take this," he said as he handed her the water and pill. "Growing older is definitely not for the faint of heart. It takes a lot of courage. Try not to worry about it."

"Well, *you're* going to worry about it if I have to buy *all new summer clothes!*" The woman squalled at him. He hugged her briefly, and she shoved him away from her.

He knew it would take a while for the calcium-magnesium-zinc to do its job, and so he simply said, "You'll figure it out," and retreated.

"*Hoh!*" she shrieked as she slammed her arms down and stomped her foot. The dogs erupted with barking at her and the commotion she created.

What Is Your Body Mass Index?

Formula – Multiply your weight in pounds by the number 703, for example: 130 pounds x 703 = 91,390. Multiply your height in inches by your height in inches, for example: 66 inches x 66 inches = 4356. Divide 91,390 by 4356 = 20.99. That is the body mass index (BMI) of a person who weighs 130 pounds and is 5-foot six-inches tall. This formula is for adults. The calculation for children is different.

Ranges of Normal to Obese – A normal body mass index is from 18.5 to 24.9. An overweight body mass index is from 25 to 30. An obese Class I body mass index is from 30.1 to 34.9. An obese Class II body mass index is from 35 to 40. An obese class III body mass index is over 40.

If your BMI is in the normal range, but you have a small amount of belly fat, you are probably okay. If you're not in the normal range, you are at risk.

Risks of Carrying Excess Belly Fat

Multiple Risks – If you carry extra belly fat, it increases your risk of heart disease or stroke, cancer, type 2 diabetes, insulin resistance, too much bad cholesterol, too little good cholesterol, metabolic syndrome, and sleep apnea.

Change in Fat Distribution – The facts are simple: when we get older our metabolism slows down, and fat increases. The fat distribution in the body changes after menopause or andropause. The arms, legs, and hips become thinner, and the middle becomes bigger. Additionally, hormonal changes could cause your body to break down and store fat differently. You could remain exactly the same weight, and still have a fatter middle. If you have a normal body mass index, but have a lot of fat around your waist, it is still unhealthy.

Hereditary – In addition to the metabolic factor, some people are predisposed to belly fat. It's hereditary.

How to Get Rid of Belly Fat

Exercise – The good news is that belly fat responds well to exercise. In fact, if you haven't been exercising, and you begin exercising now, that might be the first spot where you will notice a change. Belly fat decreases with moderate-intensity cardio exercise. If you have an obese body mass index and health issues, consult your doctor about your exercise plan. If you're healthy, get moving! Start walking briskly every day or choose another cardio activity.

Build Up Your Muscles – Muscle burns more calories, and it gives you more shape, so that you can hold your stomach in, and stand straighter.

Cut Refined Carbohydrates Out of Your Eating Plan – Stop eating white bread, pasta, and processed carbohydrates. Count the carbohydrates, and limit them to 70 grams a day, until you achieve a normal body mass index. Add the grams of carbohydrates back into your eating plan gradually. Don't consume beyond 100 grams of carbohydrates a day.

Limit Alcohol Intake – Limit yourself to no more than two glasses of wine a day. There are 7.6 grams of carbohydrates in wine, and 7.0 grams of carbohydrates in a twelve ounce can of beer. The vote is still out on whether beer gives a person a beer belly because wine can cause a person to gain weight too.

Firm Up the Stomach Muscles – 1) Lie on the floor with bent legs, and feet resting flat on the floor. 2) Sit up halfway, and extend the arms straight out in front of you on either side of your bent legs. 3) Use the stomach muscles to press your belly button down, as if you pressed it into your spine, with as much effort as possible. 4) While in that position, alternately lift your legs off the floor to a slow and deliberate count of twenty-five.

Perform fifteen of the twenty-five count sit-ups. Try to do at least five at a time before resting. Eventually, you'll be able to do all fifteen without a break.

Balance Calories Consumed and Calories Burned – Belly fat could also be caused by a simple imbalance between the amount of calories consumed, and the amount of calories burned. Cut down on your calories, and burn it off with aerobic exercise.

Presence and Posture 5

Anecdote

The man and woman walked every evening for a few miles. The woman commented, "If you don't stand up straight, pretty soon you won't be able to. You're getting a hump on your neck."

The man didn't want a permanent hump on his neck, and so he complied with the woman. Several days later he complained, "I can't feel my fingers."

"You'd better go see the doctor," she replied and lifted her eyebrows with questioning.

The man visited his doctor, and explained his malady with the fingers. The doctor examined him, and expounded, "It's probably a pinched nerve in your neck." The doctor asked the man, "What are you doing differently?"

"I'm standing up straight," answered the man.

"*Well, don't do that!*" declared the doctor.

The man and woman walked again that evening, and the man didn't make the effort to stand up straight. The woman inquired, "Can you feel your fingers?"

"Yes, if I don't try to stand up straight," he answered and smiled while he slouched and walked along gingerly. "I guess it's too late."

Posture and Self-Esteem

First Impression – The first characteristic we notice about a person when he or she walks into a room is how the person carries himself or herself. It tells the observer how the person feels about himself or herself.

Posture Improves the Waistline – Walk to a mirror, turn sideways, arch your spine slightly, and push your shoulders back. It makes a difference how trim the waistline appears. A person could look as much as five pounds lighter around the waist.

Don't Slouch – The girl's dad always had a good posture until he started to age, and then his shoulders drooped, and he slumped along when he walked. The girl started to develop the same kind of posture problem just before she came into her teen years. Many young women were embarrassed by a generous chest, and she was one of them. The girl was her full height and size, by the time she was ten years old, and so were her bosoms.

The girl was showing a 4-H calf at the Minnesota State Fair, when the cattle judge walked up to her and said, "You're a Van Dyke, aren't you? You look just like your dad, and you slouch like him too. Stand up straight when you show your animals. Show your calf with pride!" The girl's face turned bright red, she immediately straightened up, and the calf won a blue ribbon. The judge did the girl a huge favor by telling her to improve her posture. That slouch at such a young age could have stuck with her, and lasted for an entire lifetime.

Employ the Singer's Stance

How to Employ the Singer's Stance – At thirteen years of age, the young woman began voice lessons with the renowned Madame Mady, a former German Opera star. The teacher didn't allow any singing until the singer understood the singer's stance. Madame Mady told the student to part her feet so that her body balanced over them. She directed the young woman to unlock her knees to avoid fainting with stage fright. The teacher ordered the student to face her hips directly forward, and stand up straight. Madame Mady explained to the young woman that she must flatten her abdomen, and lift her chest up and out, which forced her shoulders back. Last, Madame Mady taught her to lift her chin and face straight ahead.

Improved Breath Control – Madame Mady explained that if the chest wasn't up and out, the breath control was not as effective. She illustrated that the upward position of the chest prevented tension in the abdominal wall, which interfered with the movement of the diaphragm. Madame Mady clarified that the result of good posture was that it was easier to sing beautifully, and thus gave the singer more confidence. The self-assured and poised image presented to the audience caused the listeners to receive the singer with a more positive response.

Improved Blood Circulation – Assume the singer's stance, and enjoy better health due to superior blood circulation. Practice standing proud and tall, and experience less fatigue, as well as less stress on the body.

An Imaginary String – Another reminder that Madame Mady gave the young woman was to imagine a string running through the entirety of her body, and now someone pulled up on the string, which aligned her body upward and straight. Have you ever tried balancing a book on your head? It doesn't work, unless your chin is up, and you stand erect.

The Body Language of Posture

Respectful Posture – Many years later, when the young woman competed for Dairy Princess of Minnesota, the local milk association sent her to a woman skilled in the art of etiquette. The expert explained to the dairy princess that if she didn't sit up straight, and appear attentive, she was actually engaging in conduct that appeared disrespectful to the other person. Good posture is part of the conventional rules for conduct or behavior in polite society.

Disrespectful Posture – The wife noticed business colleagues at a nearby table in the restaurant where she and her husband had dinner. The listening colleague slouched in his chair while the other colleague spoke. The body language clearly announced that the sloucher wasn't interested in what the other person said.

The wife turned away when she heard a squeal to the left of her. She spied a mother who told her daughter to sit up straight, and the daughter complained. *The mother knows that the slouch is a sign of rebellion*, thought the wife.

Attitude – Body language reveals information as to the person's attitude or current state of mind. Posture reveals if the person is bored or interested.

Causes and Effects of Poor Posture

Weakened Muscles and Repetition – Weakened muscles, repetition, and job stress are a few factors that cause poor posture. Work that requires a continual bent over position, such as gardening or factory work, also could cause posture problems. Sitting in a slouched position at a desk for several hours every day could create the hump on the neck that the man had in the anecdote.

Neck Pain – Anyone who sits at the computer for hours a day is vulnerable to neck pain, especially on the side where the hand holds the mouse.

Musculoskeletal Changes – Drivers of vehicles, who sit for hours without breaks, are also defenseless from musculoskeletal changes.

The Spine and Joints – Continued poor posture can cause spinal and joint problems. A posture with rounded shoulders and a forward thrust head position places stress on the neck. A posture where the hips tilt forward and the stomach sticks out places stress on the hip joints and lower back.

Posture Analysis

Sensory and Motor Imbalances – After the wife's leg and foot injuries, her body was completely out of balance. The husband sent her to a posture specialist, who gave her a variety of tests to determine her sensory and motor skills. The tests revealed problems with posture and balance. The analyst completed her analysis, and then printed out a book for the wife, which demonstrated how to do corrective exercises and stretches. The analyst went through each exercise with the wife to ensure that she did them correctly.

If you would like to get at the root of a posture problem, see a posture corrective specialist and straighten up.

Old Habits – Even when you achieve good posture and balance, something can happen or change that will cause the old habit to return. That is the reason why the wife continues to do the exercises.

Shoulder Brace

Desk Posture – If you slouch at your desk, try wearing a shoulder brace, and don't lean on the back of the chair. Sit forward and hook your feet on the legs of the chair to force yourself to sit up straight.

Walking Posture – Arch your spine slightly. This motion forces the shoulders backward. When you arch your back slightly, don't allow your stomach to protrude or your hips to tip forward. The abdominal muscles are responsible for holding the stomach in and preventing the forward tip of the hips. Strengthen them with abdominal exercises if you notice a problem. The stomach muscle exercises described in Chapter Three are very effective.

Postural Kyphosis

Continual slouching, whether you're young or old, could lead to a condition called Postural Kyphosis, or a hunched back. If you wait too long to correct the problem, you might need surgery, so do something about it, and correct it with a brace or physical therapy.

Posture and Confidence

The wife worked at a large company, where she was the only woman on the executive committee. Good posture served her well under the circumstances. She had to stand up to criticism and suggestions. Her erect posture sent a message to the Chairman that she was up to delivering the results. Her confident demeanor captured their respect.

Loving Affection

6

Anecdote

The man and woman arose from bed, and the man jumped into the shower. The woman knocked on the shower door, and asked the man, "*Why* are you taking a shower?"

He replied, "I have a haircut this morning."

She answered, "I thought we were going to the *nursery* this morning."

He said nothing in response, because he had agreed to go to the nursery, but he had never mentioned his haircut appointment. If he said anything at all, he probably would be in more trouble with her, and so he didn't.

She politely made breakfast for him, although she didn't look happy. She knew that she would have to go to the nursery by herself, and she would have no help with the heavy lifting.

She served his food with decorum and announced perfunctorily, "Breakfast is ready." The woman said grace as she held the man's hand, and then they ate in silence. He hid behind the newspaper, and so she arose from her chair without a word, and did the dishes.

The man didn't say anything to her because it was obvious that she was mad. When she commenced with the administering of the medicines to the two little Westies, the woman could hear her man in his office attempting to change his haircut appointment to next week, but it wasn't possible for the hairdresser.

The woman hoped to depart for the nursery before the man left for his haircut so that she could walk out of the house first and insult him by not saying good-bye, but he beat her to it.

He walked to where she worked on the dogs and cursorily kissed her on the lips, and said, "I should be home in an hour and fifteen minutes."

The woman said nothing, but watched him leave, and then wiped her mouth on her sleeve. She didn't want any part of him in that moment. She departed for the nursery by herself, parked, and pushed the heavy cart all the way up to the top of the long hill to the sago palms. She loaded four large sago palms on the cart, and skidded down the hill in her athletic shoes, as the weight of the palms threatened to turn her into a runaway disaster. She picked out four lovely hanging lobelias, added them to the cart, and then pushed it inside to pay.

The clerk asked her, "Do you need any help out to your car?"

"No, I'll be fine," she said with disdain. "I pushed that heavy cart all the way up to the top of the hill by myself to get the palms. Taking them to the car is no problem." The clerk smiled and understood the undercurrent in the woman's statement.

The woman loaded the truck with the plants, two heavy bags of potting soil, and four large bags of bark. The sweat dripped down her back and her forehead and slipped off the end of her nose. She drove home, parked the truck, and unloaded all the nursery items into the side yard. When, she had the last of the heavy items in the side yard, she spied her man carrying the hanging lobelias.

He asked contritely, "What can I do to help?"

She took him to the back yard, and pointed out what work it needed. Then she returned to pot the large palms. The sweat and strain of the work calmed her temper, and she stopped feeling angry. She walked into the house when she had finished the side yard, and retrieved two bottles of water.

She kindly handed a bottle to her man, and said without emotion, "Here's a bottle of water for you."

He replied with manners, "Thank you."

"I'll make us some lunch," she commented, and retreated.

They sat silently through lunch, and ate their sandwiches. A squirrel attempted tirelessly to get the birdseed out of a squirrel-proof bird feeder.

The woman smiled at the man and said, "Look," as she pointed at the wily upside down creature. The tension between them relieved a little more. The woman excused herself, and explained, "I have to get cleaned up." She walked their dishes into the kitchen and washed them.

The man kissed her good-bye, and left for the afternoon. The woman cleaned up and went to work in her office. The man came home, and they climbed in the car to go to dinner, since it was Friday night, date night.

He politely asked her, "Where do you want to go?"

She replied with disinterest, "I don't care. You pick." Clearly, she was only going through the motions of their date night.

He attempted to make conversation with her at dinner. She recognized his efforts, and tried her best too. They smiled and waved when they spotted the neighbors at a nearby table. She forgot about her disappointment, and enjoyed the evening. They returned home, and watched a movie on television. The time came for her to go to bed. She sat on her man's lap in his easy chair, and he cuddled her as he always did, and kissed her goodnight with extra passion. She kissed him back in return, and then stood.

She smiled at him, chuckled, and said, "If you ever want your woman to feel like a servant or a piece of furniture, listen to her plans, and then tell her that you're busy when the time comes." The man slumped in his chair and felt defeated.

A Discussion of Love and Commitment

Lilia, a seventeen-year-old opera diva, discusses love with her bodyguard boyfriend, nineteen-year-old Jim, and her other bodyguard, eighteen-year-old Derek. Following is an excerpt from the fifth book in my fictional series, *Providence: Leading of the Spirit*:

Lilia reached for Jim's powerful forearm with emotion. She loved the feel of his skin, smooth and tanned, and yet with the firmness and muscle that spoke of protection. *Jim is truly a dichotomy*, she thought, *strong and gentle at the same time*.

"I need to give some thought to how to play the part of Carmen," she said as she lifted her brows at him in question. "I'd like to hear your input."

"Tell me about the story line," Jim said and focused his attention on her with interest. At that moment, the patio door opened and Derek stepped through it holding a cup of coffee. "Good morning Derek," said Jim, "Lilia is going to fill us in on the plot for *Carmen*."

Derek sat down next to Jim and replied with one of his characteristic slow smiles, "Good, I'd like to hear it."

He's always so nice to me, Lilia thought and smiled back at Derek graciously. She began, "Carmen is a beautiful and irresistible gypsy with a fiery temper."

Derek chortled, as did Jim, who said, "So far, it's true to life."

Lilia acknowledged their joke with the lifting of one eyebrow, and continued, "Carmen woos Corporal Don Jose until he falls for her completely. He rejects his current lover, becomes involved in a mutiny against his superior officer, and joins a gang of smugglers," she explained seriously, and then intently watched their faces for a response.

"In other words, her influence ruins his life," Derek interjected knowingly as he leveled his gaze on Lilia. Lilia's neck prickled as she peered back at Derek, and immediately understood the double meaning of his statement.

She defended her position with quiet forbearance. "Your love for me *didn't* ruin your life Derek. We redirected it to a more positive source, your current love, Kuhlia," she responded with gentle caring.

"It felt like the end of the world for a period of time though," Derek said with certainty and feeling as he frowned slightly at her. "I can identify with Corporal Don Jose."

"That is a *good* thing. Maybe you can give me some advice about my role," Lilia commented openly without offense, and then smiled at him sweetly. She said, "Carmen's whims turn her love from Corporal Don Jose to Escamillo, the bullfighter. How would her change of heart make you feel Jim and Derek?" Lilia asked as she eyed them with genuine interest in their opinions.

"Well, it would make me feel vengeful, that's for certain," Jim uttered a little too quickly.

Lilia quirked her head at Jim and said, "That's interesting Jim. Would it make you feel vengeful enough to *murder* Carmen?" Lilia asked, but wasn't certain that she wanted to hear the answer.

"Yes, but I'd never react to Carmen in that way because of my beliefs," Jim answered with conviction and leveled a serious gaze at her.

Derek jumped in with knitted brows and felt incredulous as to where the plot led, "*Is that what happens?*"

"Yes," Lilia said with import, "but the question is: What kind of person *is* Carmen? Does she love *both* men, or is she a woman who constantly needs the attention of a new lover? Her famous line in the beginning of the opera is, 'Love is a rebellious bird that no one can tame. He has never known law. If you don't love me I love you, if I love you, watch yourself!'"

"I think that she loves *both* men," Derek put in. Lilia understood exactly why Derek would respond in such a way. He had a deep and abiding love for Kuhlia, and they would make each other happy, but he would never recover completely from his love and loyalty for Lilia.

"I think that she's a sociopath who always needs the stimulation of a new conquest," Jim added firmly with brilliant insight.

Lilia thoughtfully regarded the two men and their responses. She blinked, gathered the right words, and said, "Carmen is a *gypsy*. Towards the end of the opera she sings, 'Free I was born and free I will die.' *I think* that her upbringing taught her to follow her heart. I also think that she believes what her heart tells her. That is the way I'd like to play it," Lilia replied pensively as she peered at the men with a contemplative expression.

"She's a fickle pickle," Jim said accusingly and frowned at Lilia.

"Don't look at me like that Jim. We're talking about the character, not me. I could never stop loving *you*," she admonished him as her eyebrow twitched with emotion. "You may look at her and see a fickle pickle, but someone else, most likely a woman, might admire her for being strong enough to follow her heart. I have to play it *both* ways because it adds a texture of ambiguity, and makes it all the more mysterious. We want the emotion it evoked in you to come alive in the theatre," Lilia finished and reached for Jim's hand. She raised it to her mouth and kissed his knuckle. "It has nothing to do with you, my love." *There it is again*, thought Jim, *her use of the term "my love." I like it.*

He smiled at her and the corners of his eyes twinkled with humor, "I understand honey, I'll try not to get you and Carmen mixed up."

"I understand too," Derek added reflectively. "We probably don't know anyone like Carmen in our immediate friendship group, but we know that free spirits like her exist."

Lilia straightened her frame and eyed both men meaningfully as she said, "Sometimes the *free spirit* doesn't extend to *every* facet of a person's life. Sometimes the creative free spirit exists separately from the emotional free spirit," Lilia explained. Both men understood that she spoke about her relationship with Jim and her dedication to him.

"*Thank God* for that blessing," Jim replied forcefully.

"'Thank God' is right. It's His Word that gives us the guidance that we need to be happy," Lilia offered as she smiled in joyful peacefulness, "instead of running rampant in our own free will."

"I love you guys," Derek said out of nowhere. "I love who you are."

"We love who you are too Derek," she smiled and then laughed softly, "Well, I'd better get ready for rehearsal. We've slain enough dragons for one morning!" Both men stood with her and laughed. Jim opened the patio door for her, and then guided her inside with his hand placed lovingly on the small of her back. They were a couple whose steadiness tested through time.

Miss-Communication

Love *is* a rebellious bird. Think back to the tiff between the man and woman in the anecdote at the beginning of the chapter. The man didn't love the woman less. He only made a silly mistake about *when* they planned to go to the nursery. There are more ways for humans to miss-communicate with each other than blades of grass under the sun! Love conquers even such misunderstandings.

Love Is Biological and Psychological

Love is Biological – Hormones, pheromones, and neurotrophins drive physical love. When a person becomes enamored with another person, he or she often experiences a rapid heart rate or shortness of breath.

Love is Psychological – On the other hand, it is also true that brain activity increases when a person is in love, and that the person craves the love just as he or she would crave water or something to eat.

A Long-Term Commitment

Love and Commitment – As a person loves one person over an extended period, love becomes more about commitment. Love and commitment *must* grow together. When love and commitment don't grow equally, a couple often separates from each other.

Ability to Love – Love is possibly the only element that is worth living for: the ability to love someone else. God armed us with the mystical ability to love other people. It is innate. A person may feel a romantic attraction to another person, which drives the couple to mate with each other. Once they spend substantial time with each other, the individuals in the couple develop an attachment to each other. That attachment helps the couple to extend the relationship to long-term commitment.

Greatest Treatise on Love Ever Written

What Love Is – Possibly the greatest treatise ever written about love appears in the Bible in 1 Corinthians 13:

"If I speak in the tongues of men and of angels, but have not love, I am only a resounding gong or a clanging cymbal. If I have the gift of prophecy and can fathom all mysteries and all knowledge, and if I have a faith that can move mountains, but have not love, I am nothing. If I give all I possess to the poor and surrender my body to the flames, but have not love, I gain nothing"

"Love is patient, love is kind. It does not envy, it does not boast, it is not proud. It is not rude, it is not self-seeking, it is not easily angered, it keeps no record of wrongs. Love does not delight in evil but rejoices with the truth. It always protects, always trusts, always hopes, always perseveres."

"Love never fails. But where there are prophecies, they will cease; where there are tongues, they will be stilled; where there is knowledge, it will pass away. For we know in part and we prophesy in part, but when perfection comes, the imperfect disappears. When I was a child, I talked like a child, I thought like a child, I reasoned like a child. When I became a man, I put childish ways behind me. Now we see but a poor reflection as in a mirror; then we shall see face to face. Now I know in part; then I shall know fully, even as I am fully known."

"And now these three remain: faith, hope, and love. But the greatest of these is love."

Don't' Give Up – Most of us have failed on every one of these accounts at one time or another. The challenge that we face is not to give up on each other. Some families don't outpour affection on each other, and so the children learn the aloofness from their parents. If you are demonstratively affectionate, and your partner is not, teach your partner how to be more loving. We're all still learning.

The Difference between Love and Lust

Directed Inward or Outward – There is a big difference between love and lust. Lust is completely selfish and directed inwards, and love is absolute unselfishness directed outwards towards others.

Selfishness – Because we're human, love goes against our natural inclinations. Only through God are we able to love someone else and not expect anything in return. It is because of his love for us that we can take that love and translate it towards others.

Placing Others First – As we grew up, we learned manners to help us operate in the world of other people. Love is more than acting courteously or agreeing with someone's opinion. It requires effort and genuine feelings, and the conscious thought to place others first.

Love Is Visceral – Your partner's hand and the way he or she brushes your skin might touch you deeply. Most people feel highly emotional about the way their partner expresses love to him or her. A gentle touch of caring could communicate two things: strength and gentleness. Love wants to give, receive, and protect.

Love Is Healthy

Your partner's touch helps you physically. A partner's loving touch lowers the amount of cortisol released into a person's system in response to stress. Prolonged stress causes prolonged cortisol secretion, which can cause the physiological consequences that we suffer from stress. It can also weaken your immune system, and increase your blood pressure. When a person expresses love to another person, the brain releases a variety of neurotransmitters, which stimulate pleasure and can affect sleep, mood, attentiveness, memory, and the ability to learn.

Love and Ambiguity

Love is full of ambiguity. We view love differently than our mates.

The husband believed that love was patience and forgiveness. The wife knew that had to be true, since he was married to her! The wife understood her shortcomings. She knew that she was too quick to flash, and too slow to apologize. She felt thankful that her husband had the maturity to manage the two character flaws with finesse.

The wife believed that love was kindness and unselfishness. On occasion, the husband didn't bend from his will. When that happened, the wife let him have his way, and didn't make an issue of it.

Love Never Dies

"Free I was born and free I will die," sings Carmen, but love never dies. God places love in our hearts. We know that God's love is eternal. Is our love eternal too?

Growth of Love and Commitment – A man met a woman and fell passionately in love with her. His love was an undying feeling of affection characterized by strength, depth, sincerity, tenderness, devotion, loyalty, and passion. The woman accepted his love willingly and gloried in it. She thought that it would last forever, that is just how secure it felt to her, and so she lavished love on him in return. He accepted her love and they grew in love and commitment together.

A Dissipated Commitment – The years passed and one of them strayed from the path of commitment. The marriage didn't feel exciting anymore, and so the eyes wandered. Without realizing that it was even happening, one of them dissipated the commitment with an affair.

Loss of Affection Anxiety – The spouse felt the loss of the other's affection and devotion and developed anxiety about the relationship. The anxiety sought relief in the form of another love. The couple divorced and wondered how it ever happened to them. Where did the love go that each of them offered and accepted from each other?

Choice and Action – We know that love is a choice and an action, not just a feeling. A person may not feel the same passion for the other as before because he or she *chose* not to exhibit the affection anymore, but the couple *did* feel the love at one time. The special love turned to bitterness when it remembered the way it used to be, but what happened to the love that they showed to each other? Did it disappear or remain in the memory of the person who accepted it?

Internalized Love – A parent showered love upon a child. The child remembered and developed a loving nature. The child grew up into an adult, and the parent died. The child still remembered the parent's love, and it became part of who the child would always be. Does an alienated spouse remember the love too?

Love Is in the Memory – A person's memory holds the love and cherishes it even after the other person no longer offers it. Like the parent and child, that love becomes a part of whom that person will always be. It helps to explain why, even after decades, that former lovers continue to feel animosity for each other and are not comfortable talking to each other. The love that existed in the past still lives on in their hearts and memory, and has become a part of whom they are. It's hard not to feel resentment at its discontinuance. There may not be a logical reason for the resentment, but maybe that *is* the reason because *love is eternal.*

God Is Love – God is love, and therefore, so are the children of God. Our love and the love we've received must be eternal too. It's obvious that the benefits of love, whether long-term or not, far outweigh the benefits of not loving at all. Live healthy and love fully.

Sexual Intimacy

Anecdote

This anecdote is an excerpt from the second book in my fiction series, *Confidence: Reliance on the Spirit*:

Jacob began stretching his arms, shoulders, wrists, legs, and neck. He said with authority to Francine, "It's important to warm up your muscles, honey, because bowling can be strenuous. The ball is pretty heavy." He pulled his left arm all the way over to the right with his right arm.

Francine didn't want to take her eyes off Jacob as he stretched. She could see the form of every muscle as he moved them around. He looked almost as muscular as he was the day she had met him on the beach fourteen years ago. *He was a hunk back then, and he's still a hunk now*, she thought as she smiled at her good luck.

"Start stretching honey," suggested Jacob. Francine watched how Jacob did his stretches and followed suit.

Paul determined the order of play because he knew more about bowling strategy than the others. "Jacob, you go first, followed by Francine and Mary. I'll go last. Jacob, you're up," Paul smiled. He felt pleased that Jacob and Francine had decided to join their team.

Francine watched carefully as Jacob postured with the ball, and then stepped and threw it. *My, he has nice muscular legs*, Francine mused. She could see his muscles bulging through his shorts. *O-o-o-o-o-o, and when he holds the ball, look at his biceps, will you?* Silently, Francine said to herself, "*Husband, you have earned the name 'Hot Stuff.'*"

Jacob's first ball took down six pins, and his second ball took down one pin. Jacob's score remained seven for the first frame.

Francine readied herself to throw the ball. "I'm just going to take this slow and methodical," she announced to Jacob with determination. She held her ball with her feet together, pulled her arm back nice and easy, and released a slow roller.

Jacob viewed Francine's shapely curves from behind. He knew he'd better not focus on it too much, or he would embarrass himself in front of everyone. She was just about the most voluptuous woman he had ever met. Jacob smiled with pleasure. He watched as Francine's slow roller took down all ten pins.

"*Strike*, that's great Francine! Now you get your second shot *and a bonus shot! Go for it!*" Francine gave Jacob one of her magnificent full, white teeth smiles. *Man*, he reflected as he gazed at her, *that smile is enough to light up the whole room*. He looked around. Several of the other men thought so too. *I must be the luckiest man in here*, Jacob thought and grinned.

Francine delivered another slow roller. "I got another strike!" Francine jumped up and down as the team cheered for her.

Jacob observed her generous bosoms bouncing in their carriage. *M-m-m-m, I have to stop thinking about Francine in that manner*, he thought and hollered, "Keep up the good work, Francine!"

Francine delivered yet a third slow roller. This time, however, the ball only took down seven pins. "O-o-o-o-o, I'm sorry everyone. I'll try to do better next time!"

"What are you *talking* about Francine?" exclaimed Paul. "You're doing *phenomenal!* Mary, you're up next." He clapped his hands together for encouragement. "Do your thing Mary!"

Mary knocked five pins down on her first throw and the other five down on her second toss for a spare. Francine yelled and clapped "*Go Mary!*"

Jacob felt happy that Francine was having so much fun. He observed two men, who stood behind them and ogled Francine. Jacob bent and kissed Francine unexpectedly to claim his wife as his own.

"Oh Jacob dear," said Francine romantically and kissed him right back. Jacob gave the two men "the look." Now, Jacob also wished that they had a lane down near the end where no one could see Francine. He sat down and put his arm around her. *Jacob is certainly amorous tonight*, thought Francine. She smiled deliciously at him. Jacob couldn't wait to go home and get Francine into bed.

Paul was up next. *Strike! Strike! Strike!* Paul delivered a perfect score of thirty! "*Way to go, Paul, fantastic frame! Keep up the good work!*" Jacob hollered in support. They all applauded and hooted for Paul.

The evening passed quickly. Jacob's final score for the game was one-hundred-eighty. Francine's was one-hundred-ninety, a par bowler on the first try. Mary's score was one-hundred-sixty-three and Paul brought in one of the only perfect games he had ever had for a score of three-hundred. Jacob and Francine enjoyed each other's company immensely. Everyone felt the evening was a hit.

When they returned home, Jacob hurriedly prepared himself for Francine as he tore off his clothes on the way to their room. He thought about what the Bible said regarding sexual relations between married couples. He remembered what it said in Corinthians 7:4: "The wife gives authority over her body to her husband, and the husband gives authority over his body to his wife."

It had always been that way between Francine and him, even more so after their trip to Mammoth Mountain in California. They had regained some of the spontaneity that they had lost over the years.

Francine stripped off her clothes slowly and methodically just like her bowling. She stood and let Jacob appreciate her form. Next, she lowered her panties, kicked them up in the air, lied down on the bed, and stretched out her gorgeous long legs. Jacob didn't need any more invitation than that to invite him into bed. He quickly finished peeling off his clothes and dumped them on the floor. Jacob crawled into the bed next to his beauty.

"O-o-o-o-o-o-o-o, Jacob my love, you are one handsome man." She kissed his lips with a passion she couldn't remember and whispered, "*I just love bowling.*"

Physical Intimacy

Tender Touching – Men and women enjoy sexual intimacy more if there is physical intimacy first. Kiss your partner on the cheek or lips when you see him or her. Go to a movie and cuddle your partner's hand in both of your hands. Hug your partner resoundingly before departing to go somewhere. Massage your partner's neck or shoulders. Slowly, and methodically, rub your partner's feet. Hold your mate in your arms while sitting on the sofa. Allow your mate to place his or her head in your lap, and then touch the ear tenderly. To crawl into bed, and wait for the magic doesn't work for most people. We need the knowledge that our partner cares for us, that we belong to our partner.

Repetition – Unfortunately, the repetition of an activity, such as sexual intimacy, can lead to shortcuts, just like any other repeated activity. Shortcuts in an intimate encounter dilute the experience.

Trust in Each Other

Conversation – The conversation leading up to a sexual encounter is important too. Don't discuss something as joy killing as bills just before the act of intimacy.

Common Desire to Join – Each partner needs to show the other partner that he or she has the same interest in joining. It takes a lot of courage to remain vulnerable to another's needs because it could lead to disappointment. Will the other person reciprocate the pleasure that you offer? That's always a question, no matter how many years a couple has been together. People need physical closeness and eye contact when they are intimate. We need to know and have a trust in the other person.

Intimacy Is Healthy

Release of Neurotransmitters – Physical intimacy causes your brain to release the pleasure-stimulating neurotransmitters of oxytocin, dopamine, and serotonin, and reduces the stress hormone of cortisol in your body. Oxytocin helps a person to bond and build trust with another person. Sex can improve your sense of smell, increase your immunity, and help to lower your blood pressure. Stressful feelings of loneliness can accompany a lack of physical intimacy. Sexual intimacy stabilizes a relationship. Sex is good for you!

Emotional Bonding – Sexual intimacy increases your emotional bond to your mate. The value of sex in a relationship has evolved past reproduction. It is essential to the creation and maintenance of a strong emotional bonding. The ability to love another person is one of the greatest gifts that God gave to us as human beings.

Caring Encourages Intimacy

Try to Please – Think back to when you first met your significant other. Do you remember how hard you tried to ensure his or her happiness? Has this endeavor lost importance? If the way to your partner's heart is through his or her stomach, use it! Make the effort to prepare a nice meal for him or her. If your partner enjoys a good movie, go to one.

Affection Dispels Insecurities – As we grow older, insecurities creep into a relationship, but affection dispels them. Hug your partner in the morning right after you get out of bed to remind him or her of how much your love for each other means to you. Kiss your partner goodbye before you leave to go somewhere. Affectionately hold your partner's hand.

Stand Up for Your Partner – When a member of the family picks on your partner, choose the side of your partner. Don't focus on the troublemaker's thoughts or motivations. Make that your personal policy, to stand together as a team. There isn't anything sexier than that. It proves more than any other factor that you love your partner, and it makes your partner desire to love you in return.

Romance

Remember the special moments, and what caused them to be romantic. Revisit those times occasionally to give your relationship a shot of fresh air. Here is a true story to demonstrate a special moment of romance:

In 1980, the woman visited Oahu to meet a girlfriend returning from China. She and her girlfriend walked through the village of the hotel, and looked in the jewelry stores. A man watched them from outside the store's window.

The next day, the girlfriend and the woman soaked in some sun on the beach. They had beach mats, and so did the man from the night before. When the women decided to swim, he decided to swim. When the women moved their mats to the shadows of the palms, he positioned his mat in the shadow of the palms. When the women moved back into the sun, he also moved back into the sun. It was comical, and the girlfriend and the woman laughed about it.

The girlfriend said within his earshot, "I'd like to get a Mai-Tai."

The woman answered, "A diet coke sounds good to me." They arose from their mats, and then the woman turned to the man and said, "Well, are you coming too?" He shook his head up and down enthusiastically, and that is how the woman met her husband of thirty years.

∞

Probably, every one of you has one infamous place, which lightens your mood, and gives you pleasure, a location where you first fell in love. Stay in touch with the feelings that you had back then, and plan another visit to your magical location.

The Bond of Intimacy

The bond of intimacy displays itself in an interpersonal attraction. This anecdote demonstrates the connection:

The wife felt so close and content with the husband's company that she had no need or desire to be apart from him. They did almost everything together. The wife thought the husband was truly funny, like no other man whom she knew, and it tickled her.

They went to dinner on their date night. The hosts stood right next to the couple's table and organized the availability of the tables around them.

One young woman called out the numbers, "*Seventy-one, eighty-six, ninety-three!*"

The husband quickly and quietly said in the wife's ear, "I hope those are the numbers of the tables and not our ages!"

The wife laughed hilariously, and felt a deep-seated emotional bond with her husband. It had no other logical outlet than intimacy.

Prostate Cancer

Anecdote

The woman returned home from UCLA where she studied cellular metabolism and molecular genetics with a class of doctor interns. She didn't even know why she had taken the course, but tonight was the last night, and she had aced it. She climbed into bed next to the man. She could tell that there was something wrong. The man's head drooped, and a tear slid down his cheek. She became alarmed, because she had only seen him cry on one other occasion, his uncle's funeral. It took a lot to move him to that state.

She brushed her hand across his forehead, and asked with deep empathy and emphasis, *"What's wrong? Did someone die?"*

He gazed at her fearfully, and felt a huge sense of loss at losing her. He was reluctant to tell her about the problem because he was older than she was, and he didn't want the problem to place an undue burden on her. He shook his head back and forth and disinclined to reply.

"Please honey, I can't help you until you tell me what's wrong!" She declared with emotion, and her eyes filled with tears too.

The fear and trepidation on his face frightened her. He turned to her and began, but his voice cracked. He started again and stared at her intently begging for understanding, "I have prostate cancer," he said as he burbled with emotion.

Suddenly, it dawned on her why she had taken the class at UCLA. She had learned everything a person needed to know about prostate and breast cancer, and what to do to help the person who has it.

Her response sounded flip and a little too confident, "No problem, I have it covered. I know what to do!"

His head popped up and he looked at her curiously and inquired, "You do?"

"Yup, that's what I studied for the last three months!" She cried with assurance.

Her answer was so surprising that the man couldn't talk right away. He finally found his tongue and offered, "I have to explore my options."

"Yes, I know honey. Don't worry, you don't have to go through this alone," she said and hugged him close to her.

Ninety-Seven Percent of Men with Prostate Cancer Survive

Vicious or Less Invasive – The wife knew two men with prostate cancer, one lived, and one died. They were the two most important men in her life, her dad, and her husband. They told her of their maladies within a few days of each other.

Her dad's prostate cancer was vicious and fast growing, and so her dad opted to have the prostate removed immediately.

Her husband's prostate cancer was growing slowly, and was less invasive. Her husband researched his options, and decided on conformal radiation. It was a heavy decision for the husband to make because the doctor informed him that if he had conformal radiation, he wouldn't be able to have surgery afterwards, even if he needed it.

Rising PSA Count After Surgery – A year after the wife's dad had his prostate removed, the doctor said that her dad should have radiation because his PSA count was rising. Her dad had the radiation and lived for another eight years, until the doctor, and he could no longer keep the PSA count under control. The cancer metastasized to the bone, and the doctor pronounced her dad terminal with two months to live.

In fact, he lived for another five months, and then succumbed to the awful disease. When he died, he had an unheard of PSA count of two thousand! The doctor told the wife that he had never seen a PSA count of two thousand in another patient in his life. The pastor at church explained to the wife that when a person has a spiritual revival, it often extends a person's life beyond what is expected.

Percentage of Men with Prostate Cancer – The professor at UCLA told the wife's class that every man would eventually get prostate cancer if he lived long enough. Many men have prostate cancer, and are completely unaware of it. Others die from something else when they've had prostate cancer for years. The wife's husband lived on with a healthy prostate, and so can you if you catch it early enough.

What is PSA?

Prostate-Specific Antigen (PSA) is a protein inside the prostate gland. If a man is normal, the protein appears in small amounts. If there is something wrong, such as prostate cancer or an enlarged prostate, the protein appears in higher amounts. A simple blood test can determine the protein amount. Even though the test is not always accurate, it's still one of the most efficient methods to determine risk.

Metastatic Prostate Cancer

High PSA – If the PSA becomes extremely elevated, as with the wife's dad, it is a strong indicator that the patient has metastatic prostate cancer. In the dad's case, it moved to his bones, but it could also move to the lymph nodes.

Advanced Prostate Cancer – In advanced prostate cancer, the cancer moves to tissue near the prostate.

Recurrence – Prostate cancer can also reoccur, whether the cancer is in the prostate or another part of the body, such as the bones or lymph nodes.

Doctor Examination

The doctor will conduct a digital rectal exam and a biopsy if he is suspicious of prostate cancer. If the patient has had prostate cancer previously, the doctor might order a bone scan, an MRI, or a CT scan. He also might do a urine flow study, which helps to pinpoint an enlarged prostate. A cystoscope, a microscope, inserted into the bladder through the urethra allows the doctor to view the problem.

Annual PSA Test for Men over Fifty

Because there are often no accompanying symptoms, every man over the age of fifty should have an *annual* PSA test. Don't take the risk of not having the PSA test.

Symptoms of Prostate Cancer

If the man does have symptoms, they might include frequent trips to the bathroom during the night, difficulty with the urine stream, burning during urination, possible blood in the urine, and an uncomfortable pain and stiffness in the area of the upper thighs, hips, and lower back.

False PSA Reads

False Positive Read – If an elevated PSA level ends in a false positive read, it could mean the man has other circumstances: a prostate infection, a recent ejaculation, an irritation of some kind (prostatitis), or benign prostatic hyperplasia (BPH), an enlarged prostate gland. Because the prostate gland surrounds the urethra, the enlarged prostate could put pressure on the urethra, and make urination more difficult.

Aging – As a man grows older, the average normal range of PSA increases.

What Problems Could Prostate Cancer Cause?

Erectile Dysfunction – Prostate cancer could cause erectile dysfunction, difficulties during sexual intercourse, problems with urination, and general pain. Most of these problems are treatable. Talk to your doctor about the side effects.

Solutions for Erectile Dysfunction – Varieties of new solutions address the erectile dysfunction problem, such as gadgets, devices, modern medicines, supplements, and implants. With all these choices, most couples can find something to improve their situation and allow them to resume a normal sexual relationship.

Treatment of Prostate Cancer

Method of Management – If you find one day that you have prostate cancer, you'll need to do your research too. The method of management varies with the individual. If the man is older, and the tumor is growing slowly, watchful waiting might be the right choice.

You have the following choices: surgery, radiation therapy, high-intensity focused ultrasound (HIFU), chemotherapy, oral chemotherapeutic drugs, positron emission tomography, cryosurgery, hormonal therapy, or a combination of the treatments mentioned. Almost all the treatments have side effects such as erectile dysfunction and urinary incontinence.

Life Choices – Sit down and talk everything over with your doctor and partner. What life changes can you tolerate? How is your general health? Consult *several* physicians, and become knowledgeable about every treatment, and the after-effects that they cause. The choice of treatment has to be right for you. Conduct meticulous research. You are the one who has to live with the choice you make.

What Should I Eat?

Don't Eat Red Meat and Dairy – Reduce or eliminate red meat and dairy from your eating plan. Processed red meats have nitrates added to it to preserve the meat's color. The body takes the nitrates and converts them to nitrosamines in the digestive tract. Nitrosamines are carcinogens, and carcinogens cause cancer.

Fruits and Vegetables – Eat as many fruits and vegetables with fiber as you can to drag the fat out of your system. Eat broccoli, cauliflower, and other cruciferous vegetables, which are high in vitamin C and fiber content. Cruciferous vegetables contain nutrients, which fight cancer in prostate cells.

Drink Green Tea – Green tea is an antioxidant that is twenty times more active than Vitamin C. It is also a powerful anticarcinogenic that inhibits cancer cells. Components in green tea actually block the growth of cancer cells, and promote the death of them.

Vitamin B6, Selenium, Vitamin E, Lycopene, and Soy – To reduce your risk of cancer, ensure that you have Vitamin B6, Selenium,

Vitamin E, Lycopene, and Soy in your nutritional plan. Ready-to-eat cereals are rich with Vitamin B6, especially Quaker Oats, which has 22 milligrams of Vitamin B6 in one serving. Quaker Oats and ready-to-eat cereals are also rich with Vitamin E. Eat nuts, mollusks, pork, and lamb, which have a high Selenium content. Eat anything made from tomatoes for Lycopene. Eat foods rich with soy such as edamame beans, soy milk, tofu, and whole soybeans.

The Value of Vitamin D

Vitamin D Deficiency – A low Vitamin D level in the blood and cancer are directly related. People who live in northern states and countries, who don't get as much sunlight, have a much greater risk of contracting and dying from cancer. If you look at the entire population in the world, more than half of the people are deficient in Vitamin D.

Sunshine and Supplements – Get out into the sunshine for fifteen minutes every day between mid-morning and mid-afternoon. Don't wear sunscreen because it blocks the UVB radiation that promotes the production of Vitamin D in your skin. Take a Vitamin D supplement of 2000 IU a day or more.

Exercise and Reduced Risk of Prostate Cancer

The general relationship between physical activity and a decreased risk of cancer is quite convincing. Dated prostate cancer and exercise studies were uncertain, but new studies show a positive relationship between exercise and reduced risk of prostate cancer. Older men should exercise vigorously at least three hours a week. The exercise reduces his risk of contracting advanced prostate cancer, or dying from the disease by seventy percent.

Breast Cancer in Women and Men

Anecdote

The woman visited the famous Minnesotan doctor at the Mayo Clinic. Another doctor had diagnosed her with endometrial cancer, and a mammogram exposed over two hundred lumps in her breasts. The woman was twenty-seven years old, a young candidate for cancer, but she had never had any children, which placed her in a higher risk group.

The doctor inquired, "Do you live on a farm?"

"I don't live on a farm now, but I grew up on a dairy farm," she answered and wondered why that question was relevant.

"Did you eat a lot of beef and dairy?" He asked her perfunctorily.

"Yes," the woman responded, "and I still do."

"Well, that's going to have to change," he replied and looked at her directly in the eyes to perceive how she felt about the new information.

"Why is that doctor?" She inquired.

"The answer is that fat in your diet increases the production of estrogen, which only fuels tumor growth," he said quietly, but firmly.

"What should I eat?" She asked him, and then listened intently.

"You should eat a low-fat diet with plenty of fruits and vegetables. For now, we're going to take you off of beef and dairy, and prescribe a diet of chicken and fish," he said as he made the notes on his chart.

She loved beef and dairy because she had grown up on them, but her condition was serious enough for her to have a life-changing reality check. She answered softly, "Okay doctor."

"Do you get a lot of exercise?" He asked her pointedly.

"I get a lot of exercise lifting, but I don't really sweat from it," she replied truthfully.

"From now on, I want you to walk, jog, run, hike, ride a bike, swim, play tennis or racquetball, or do aerobics five times a week, *or more* for forty-five minutes a session," he declared with certainty.

"Why is exercising important?" She asked him, ever curious about medical technology.

"It's important because it improves your immune system, and decreases the production of estrogen," he reported to her with conviction.

"I understand doctor. I guess I'll have to change my schedule around," She responded with indubitable confidence.

"Good, *your health* has to be your number one priority, even before earning money. Can you make that commitment?" He asked her with emphasis as he gazed at her seriously.

She straightened up in her chair, and said with determination, "Aye, aye doctor."

He chuckled, "Besides, it will put you in a better mood, help you to look amazing, and boost your self-esteem."

She smiled along with him, and chortled, "Then I won't have to ask my husband, 'Does my butt look fat in these jeans?'"

He laughed at her alacrity, and directed her, "Come to see me in six weeks after you've had the hysterectomy, and we'll see how you are doing with the lumps in your breasts."

"Yes doctor," she replied and felt encouraged by the number of ways that she could take control of her own life.

The woman thought back on that conversation, which had taken place thirty-three years ago, and marveled at how it had changed her life. Exercise and nutrition had become her focus for all the ensuing years, and it still held priority for her today. *In fact, she thought, it's every bit as important.* The doctor's methods had been controversial back in the 1970s, but she suspected that he knew he was right, even though he had died many years ago.

The woman had had the hysterectomy, followed a regimented exercise and nutrition plan, and the many lumps in her breasts had dissolved and disappeared. She was sixty years old and cancer-free.

Recently, her young doctor had given her a physical, and announced cheerily, "Continue to do whatever you're doing. You have the body of a twenty-two-year-old woman."

The woman sat in her back yard eating dinner, and enjoyed watching the birds eating from the bird feeders. She smiled to herself, and said softly, "Thank you, Doctor."

The famous doctor smiled from his perch among the clouds, and whispered, "You're welcome."

Men Get Breast Cancer Too

No man wants to hear this, but it is true. The Breast Cancer Research Foundation (BCRF) reports that doctors diagnose breast cancer in approximately 1,700 men each year. Out of that group, around 450 of those men die from the disease because of the lack of early detection. The BCRF suggests that men perform self-examinations too.

Worldwide Incidence of Breast Cancer

Percent of Cancers in Women – Breast cancer comprises over ten percent of all the cancers reported in women. It is the fifth most common cause of death from cancer. That statistic should get our attention.

Caucasian Women – Breast cancer is more common in Caucasian women than in Latina, Asian, or African-American women.

What Are the Risks?

Use of Alcohol – Alcohol increases the likelihood that a person will contract breast cancer. A higher consumption of alcohol means a greater risk of breast cancer because alcohol is a carcinogen to humans. The U.S. Department of Health and Human Services listed alcohol as a known carcinogen in humans for the first time in May of 2000.

Birth Control Pills – The use of birth control pills beyond a period of ten years also increases the risk, if the woman is under the age of thirty-five years.

Relatives – If you have a mother, grandmother, sister, or daughter diagnosed with breast cancer, your risk is also higher. That risk increases if the woman was under the age of forty when the cancer occurred.

Menstrual Cycle – An early menstrual cycle, before the age of twelve, increases the risk level.

No Children – Women with no children, or who had their children after the age of thirty, are at greater risk.

Late Perimenopause – The risk increases when the onset of perimenopause does not occur until the age of fifty-five or older.

Cancer Genes – Presence of the BCRA1 or BCRA2 gene can change your risk of contracting breast cancer in your lifetime from twelve to sixty percent. Its presence also gives you a fifteen to forty percent chance of ovarian cancer in your lifetime. The good news is that not more than ten percent of patients have these mutated genes.

Breast Cancer in One Breast – Occurrence of Breast Cancer in one breast increases the risk that a woman will have cancer in the other breast.

Obesity – Women who maintain a normal body mass index (BMI) for the entirety of their lives have less risk than those who gain weight. The risk for being overweight doubles the chances that a woman will contract breast cancer after menopause.

Diethylstilbestrol (DES) – Buy organic foods whenever possible. The beef and poultry industries used a hormone called diethylstilbestrol (DES) in the 1960s. DES causes breast cancer, and cancer of the reproductive organs. Supposedly, the use of DES discontinued by the 1970s, but there are many who disagree, and claim that its use is still prevalent in the meat sold in the United States.

What Can I Do to Lower the Risks?

Exercise – Exercise at a moderate level for forty-five minutes at least five or more days a week. Exercise boosts your immune system, and lowers the production of estrogen.

Avoid Fat – Eat plenty of fruits and vegetables, and stay away from high-fat foods. Foods with a high fat content cause a woman to produce more estrogen, which only provides more fuel to make a tumor grow.

Self-Examination – Examine your breasts at least once a month. If you discover a lump, visit your doctor immediately, even though the majority of lumps are non-cancerous. Look for changes in the way the breast looks and feels, such as the shape or texture. Notice any discharge from a nipple. Go to the Breast Cancer Research Foundation website, and look at the pictured examples. That will be enough to motivate you to conduct a monthly self-examination!

Regular Mammograms – If you're in a higher risk category, you should have an annual mammogram starting at the age of thirty-five.

Diagnosis

Detection – A medical practitioner employs three different tests to detect the presence of breast cancer: breast examination, a mammogram, and Fine Needle Aspiration and Cytology (FNAC). A general practitioner can perform the FNAC in his office. The GP uses a local anesthetic to numb the area before he or she withdraws fluid from the lump. If the fluid is clear, it is probably not breast cancer, only a benign lump. If the fluid is bloody, the GP sends it out for examination under a microscope.

Removal – The doctor also might choose to remove part of the lump, a core biopsy, or remove the entire lump, an excisional biopsy.

Stages of Cancer and Treatments

Stages of Cancer – There are five stages of cancer from Stage 0 to Stage IV. The treatment for each stage is dependent on the size of the tumor, and whether it has spread to other tissues or not.

Treatment for Stages 0 and I – In Stage 0, the treatment may be as simple as a lumpectomy. In Stage I, the cancer is no bigger than an inch. A lumpectomy also could take care of this stage, and possible radiation or chemotherapy.

Treatment for Stages II and III – In Stages II and III, the cancer has either spread to auxiliary underarm lymph nodes, or is a larger tumor, which hasn't spread to the lymph nodes. Treatment of these stages includes a lumpectomy or mastectomy, possible lymph node removal, possible radiation, and chemotherapy.

Management for Stage IV – In Stage IV, the cancer has spread to other organs, such as the liver, lungs, brain, skeletal system, or lymph nodes near the collarbone. This stage of cancer is not curable. Treatment manages the disease only. Treatment might include surgery, radiation, chemotherapy, and other targeted therapies, which will increase the patient's survival for about six months.

Breast Cancer Research Foundation (BCRF) – For specific information, go to the Breast Cancer Research Foundation, and look at the gradations for each stage of cancer.

Emotional Impact

Cancer Support Groups – Cancer is a highly emotional experience. The world has taught us to react to the word "cancer" with shock. Shock has health ramifications too, such as depression, sense of loss, preoccupation with your spouse's reaction, uncertainty, and loss of self-esteem. Thankfully, many hospitals have cancer support groups, and you can find cancer support groups on the web too.

Attitude – The woman's doctor sent her to a psychiatrist to help change her "all is lost" attitude. The psychiatrist helped her a lot by telling her, "Yes, you will be dead in six months if you don't develop a positive attitude." Her reaction to his statement was to look up to her Maker, and turn the problem over to him to reduce her amount of preoccupation with the disease.

Count Your Blessings – A few years ago, a girlfriend of mine was dying from breast cancer at the age of fifty-seven. I wrote to her to encourage her. She wrote me back just a few days before she died, and this is what the note said:

"Hi Peggy,

Thanks so much for the card and the thoughts and prayers. They are always appreciated. I'll always remember our horse talks, and Guernseys versus Holsteins (cows). We've been blessed with a beautiful fall, which I am enjoying, and I'm trying to live each day well. I know I've been blessed with wonderful long-time friends.

Love,

Liz"

As I entered the words of her note into the computer for you to read, the tears dripped down to my chin. I was especially touched by, "and I'm trying to live each day well." That seems like good advice for all of us.

Depression 10

Anecdote

The woman had had a horrible week. She came from a very large family with second and third start marriages, and it seemed like no one was getting along. Even though the woman's home was two thousand miles away from most of them, the quibbling upset her. She felt quite certain that her family thought her life was easy and comfortable because she didn't complain to her family about her woes. She didn't want to burden them, but they didn't do her the same favor. The woman sat alone in the backyard, and sipped on a white wine spritzer of her own making. She watched the palm tree branches move with the breeze, and thought about the attacks she had borne with grace that week. She felt defeated. She sighed deeply, walked upstairs, climbed into bed, and pulled the covers up over her head.

The man shook her to wake her, "I thought that we were going to the movie."

"Okay give me a few moments to get ready," she replied sleepily.

The man waited patiently, and asked her when she appeared, "Are you ready?"

"I'm ready," she responded sulkily.

"Let's go then," he said as he gazed at her with concern. "You probably just need to get out of the house."

She nodded glumly, but didn't add anything else. The man parked the car, and helped her out of the car. He took her hand and led her down the sidewalk. He bought himself a treat while she found them two seats all the way in the back of the theater. She sat through the entire movie with very little interest. When the movie was over, the man again took her hand and led her back to the car. She said nothing. When they arrived at home, she immediately returned upstairs and again climbed into bed. She slept in escape of the problems that burdened her. She slept all night, and through the next day and night. She stayed in bed for two days without getting up to do dishes, laundry, or any other household chores.

The man said on the third morning, "I wish you'd try to shake this depression off. Aren't you hungry?"

"No, I'm not hungry. Exercise will help. I think I'll have a good workout," she rolled out of bed, and could barely walk to the dressing room.

She forced herself to dress in exercise clothing, and approached the recumbent bicycle. She sat down, programmed it, and purposely took off at a brisk pace. The sweat poured off her brow, and dripped from her forehead, even into her ears. Soon she felt a little better as the endorphins kicked in, and her spirit rose a little.

The man walked upstairs, and asked her, "When is the last time you took SAM-e?"

"I don't remember," she replied.

"You have to make SAM-e your *highest* priority. You can't afford to forget it," he said as he reprimanded her gently. He handed her a tablet, and a glass of water. "Here," he said.

"I know that it is important. You're right. I'll try not to forget again," she panted, as she accepted the pill.

"Good," he answered and kissed her on the cheek. "I'm happy to see you out of bed," he smiled at her. "How do you feel?"

"I wish you wouldn't perpetually ask me that question," she said with slight angst.

"I know, I know. I won't ask you anymore," He replied and smiled at her again. It was good to see her go back to her regular routine.

Stress Responses in Different Individuals

Expectations – All people have chronic problems, even those that don't manifest or talk about their problems. How does one person get through divorce, death, or loss of a job without a depression episode, and another person does not? Much of it has to do with a person's expectations, but there's more.

Feelings of Hopelessness – The young woman's dad optimistically developed a huge and successful farm, until he and her mom divorced, and he had to split everything in half. His depression became so acute that he slept on the sofa every available moment of the day. He didn't watch television, didn't enjoy a good steak, couldn't remember anything, displayed extreme irritability, and generally felt a hopelessness that conquered him. It made the young woman so sad at the time because he turned into a completely different person. The depression lasted for a couple of years, until he auctioned off everything, moved to northern Minnesota, and started all over again. He got through it, but it was a difficult and arduous process. He married a woman with an upbeat personality, which seemed to improve his mood tremendously.

Move On with Your Life – The woman's husband lost his job as a senior executive for a Fortune 500 company when the company had a reduction in force and let thousands of people go. He made the lists of those that were about to lose their jobs, but didn't realize that another list existed, which included him and his boss. His response was to move forward quickly, and find another way to make a living. He networked and took work, wherever he could get it. He took over the woman's formal dining room as his office. He became an international business consultant, and traveled across the world without a complaint to anyone.

Biological, Psychological, and Learned Factors – If something like the two above events happened to the young woman, it sent her into a depression so deep that it took weeks, and sometimes months for her to cycle out of it. The young woman was her father's daughter, and it occurred to her that her depressed state might be biological, and not just psychological, or she thought she might have socially learned it from her dad. In truth, all three of these factors determine a person's response to stress.

Exercise Improves Mood

Exercise Decreases Depression – The lack of energy caused by the depression threatens to defeat us, but we can't let it because exercise helps. The neurotransmitters and endorphins released during exercise provide a natural mood elevator. Exercise decreases the production of cortisol, which can weaken your immune system, and increase your blood pressure. Exercise raises body temperature, which has a calming effect on the body.

Exercise and Control of Your Life – When everything around you is spinning out of control, exercise is something that you can control. It is a positive response to a horrible situation, instead of a negative response, such as giving up. Exercise causes our brains to focus on something else besides the problem, and thus gives us temporary relief from the problem. The movement causes us to feel better about ourselves because exercise is good for us, which means that we have made the right choice.

Build Movement into Your Day – Exercise is movement. Exercise can be accomplished through an organized program, or working on the tasks that need attention on your property. Let the gardener go, or reduce his tasks, so that you can take up the slack and work outside. Living plants and nature provide an uplifting environment for a depressed spirit. Forget about the car wash, retrieve the hose, and do it yourself. Surprise your dog, and take the loving creature on an unexpected walk around the block. It will make you pet happy, and help your mindset as well.

Use a break at work to walk around the building or the block. Take your refreshment with you. When you return to work, take the stairs instead of the elevator. When you go to lunch off the property, park your car at the far end of the parking lot so that you can walk before and after lunch. Regular movement helps to manage severe depression.

Amount of Exercise Needed

Thirty minutes of moderate-intensity exercise five or more days a week helps to address extended depression. It also considerably lowers the risks of obesity, diabetes, cardiovascular disease, and some types of cancers.

The Nutritional Supplement, SAM-e (S-Adenosylmethionine)

Regain Control of Your Life – SAM-e is a miraculous supplement, which helps with joint function, energy, liver function, *and* brain function. It is a natural mood enhancer because it supports the proper function of the neurotransmitters in the brain. It is the most important substance to brain metabolism. Within a few minutes, you will notice the difference. If you have severe depression, take the full dose daily, and don't allow depression to defeat you. SAMe comes packaged in foil, and for a reason. It loses its potency and effectiveness quickly after removed from the packaging, so don't punch it out until you're ready to pop it into your mouth.

Melatonin – The Sleep Hormone

Lack of Sleep and Depression – A bad night's rest can destroy a person's sense of humor in short order. Ongoing nights without enough rest often result in depression.

Unsynchronized Day-Night Clock – People who suffer from depression could have a melatonin production cycle, which is out of synchronization. If a person has high levels of melatonin in their blood when they wake in the morning, their melatonin day-night cycle might have switched at some point. High levels of melatonin in the blood should occur later in the day. Exposure to bright light in the morning encourages the natural production of melatonin later in the day. Take a walk in the sunshine or get exposure to bright light in the morning to change the clock back.

Less Melatonin Production with Age – As we age, our bodies produce less melatonin. An older person might not produce any melatonin anymore. A melatonin supplement before bedtime helps with this problem. If you have any medical concerns, consult your doctor.

Sun and Serotonin

Production of Serotonin – Our brains produce more of the natural mood-lifting chemical, serotonin, on a sunny day than on a cloudy day. Too many dark days can lead to Seasonal Affective Disorder (SAD) in people living in gloomy climates. Being in the sunshine always helps a person to feel better, not to mention the beneficial connection between Vitamin D and the prevention of certain types of cancers.

Sunning Routine – The wife and the husband had an upstairs front porch, which faced the street. Their two Westies spent the bulk of their day on the porch until the couple finished working. Even on the coldest days, the dogs spread out in the sunshine, and returned inside panting from the warmth. The wife wondered about the temperature in the middle of winter, and decided to try it for herself. It was very pleasant. She bought herself a cushioned rug, and decided to hang out with the dogs!

Adjusting the Routine from Summer to Winter – After her exercise routine, the wife slipped into her bikini and headed for the porch. Fifteen minutes on the front side, and fifteen minutes on the backside satisfied her need for the sun. The amount of time she spent on the porch varied from winter to summer. When the sun was in apogee, orbiting the furthest from the earth, she added a few more minutes. When the sun was in perigee, orbiting the closest to the earth, she decreased the number of minutes. If the wife skipped too many days in a row, she could tell the difference in her mood. The husband usually directed the wife back out to the porch if her mood dipped. He was a good husband, but also knew how to protect himself!

Sun Availability – If you live in a wintry climate, survey your home to find out when and where the sun is available to you. Consider converting a room into a solarium. Get outside into the sunshine whenever you can. Change your environment so that more light can enter.

Seasonal Affective Disorder – If your doctor has diagnosed you with Seasonal Affective Disorder, you could purchase a light therapy screen, which produces light similar to sunlight. Your mood will lift with exposure to light.

Menopause

Anecdote

The man and woman celebrated their twenty-fifth wedding anniversary. The man took the woman to their mountain retreat in the High Sierra Nevada Mountains for a special weekend. He made a reservation for dinner at the super-exclusive Lakefront Restaurant on Twin Lakes.

The woman dressed for the dinner in black jeans, a crisp white blouse, and a red leather coat to compensate for the cool evening. She straightened her long blonde hair, and wore it down tucked behind her ears. She meticulously applied her cosmetics, and smiled in the mirror. Last, she fastened a heavy turquoise necklace around her neck, and a matching bracelet and ring on her right wrist and ring finger. She pulled on her red cowboy boots, and felt satisfied with her appearance. She didn't want her husband to think that he wasn't worth dressing up for anymore. He was more precious to her today than he had ever been.

The zephyrs kicked up and lowered the evening temperatures considerably more for a midsummer night. The woman wrapped a scarf around her neck to protect her from the breezes, and the couple headed out for their destination.

The wintry summer evening didn't daunt the couple even though the restaurant didn't have heat in the summertime. The woman kept her red jacket on, and perused the menu, as did the man. He thought he should praise the woman on how lovely she looked this evening. He noticed the effort that she had made to look stunning for him, and so did everyone else when the couple first entered the restaurant. He glanced up at the woman to tell her.

Her face, ears, and neck turned bright red, and now matched her jacket. "Oh dear I'm flashing!" She cried and quickly removed her jacket and scarf, pulled her long hair off her neck, and tried to recuperate.

The makeup on her forehead dripped, and carried a stream of it through her blush down to her chin. She grabbed a napkin and dabbed at her face as the sweat poured into her ears and onto her crisp white blouse, which turned blotchy with dark spots as the sweat continued. The woman took off her necklace and bracelet, and shoved them into her purse. She used the scarf to tie her hair away from her neck and face. She quickly retrieved a tissue from her purse and wiped her face with it. The mascara dripped past her cheekbones while she attempted to manage it. She hurriedly pushed her socks down and slipped off her cowboy boots under the table.

The lovely woman morphed into a clown face right before the man's eyes. The man tried not to break out into laughter, but smirked at her with large round eyes of surprise instead.

The waiter approached their table, and asked, "Are you ready to order?"

The woman peered at the man meaningfully, and he replied for them, "Give us a moment."

The waiter glimpsed at the woman, and wondered what her

problem was. She had appeared so gorgeous when they first arrived, and now she had no makeup, and had disrobed as far as decently proper in a restaurant. The man didn't compliment her on her appearance, but watched her discomfiture with humor.

He said quietly, "Thank you for dressing for me this evening honey."

"You're welcome dear," the woman replied as she pulled off her leather belt and pulled the shirt out of her pants. The diners in the restaurant peered at her curiously. A middle-aged woman at another table laughed openly. The woman hung her tongue out like a dog and panted, as she declared, "Perimenopause is not for the faint of heart."

"Take heart," the man responded. "It should be over soon."

"That's not what the doctor told me," answered the woman with chagrin. "He said that it could last into my sixties! Just imagine thirteen years of this!"

The man laughed outright at her complete exasperation, and commented, "Maybe you should wear a swimsuit under your clothes."

"No one likes a smart you know what," snapped the woman with indignation. The diners in the intimate little restaurant chuckled at the comical scene and shook their heads with amusement.

What are Menopause, Perimenopause, Postmenopause, and Premenopause?

Menopause – In women with their uterus, menopause is not just the cessation of the menses, it is also the cessation of the reproductive hormones in the ovaries. In women without a uterus, it is the cessation of the reproductive hormones by a remaining ovary. Doctors can identify the approach of menopause by very elevated levels of follicle stimulating hormones (FSH). Menopause doesn't officially occur until the cessation of the menses for twelve months after the last menstrual bleed.

Perimenopause – This is the span of time before complete cessation of the menses, or the ovaries stop production of reproductive hormones. Some women reported a perimenopause that continued for thirteen or more years. The reason for the extended years of discomfort is that the symptoms often begin before and continue after perimenopause.

Postmenopause – In women with a uterus, postmenopause commences with the cessation of the menses for twelve months. In women without a uterus, postmenopause begins by the identification of very elevated levels of the follicle stimulating hormones (FSH).

Premenopause – In women with a uterus, this is the time before any irregularities occur in the menses. In women without a uterus, this is the time before the woman experiences any perimenopause symptoms.

What Are the Symptoms of Perimenopause?

Different for Everyone – The symptoms vary from woman to woman. Some women, who have had several children, don't experience any symptoms worth noting. Other women, who have not had children, experience some of the worst meltdowns possible. The rapidly fluctuating levels of hormones cause a number of discomforts.

Hot Flashes or Flushes – At the beginning of perimenopause, a woman might experience as many as sixteen to twenty major duty hot flashes a day. Night sweats might persistently soak her nightgown, hair, and bedding and disrupt her sleep. Towards the end of perimenopause, the flashes occur less, for example, a woman might only have one hot flash each morning before arising.

A hot flash or flush is caused by a sudden rise in a woman's body temperature, which reaches the higher temperature very quickly. The flash occurs when the body temperature is slow to return to normal. The occurrence of the flash can cause a woman to sweat profusely or feel weak.

Moodiness, Anxiety, and Irritability – A hot flash like the one described in the anecdote can cause a rapid mood swing. The rapidly fluctuating levels of reproductive hormones can cause a woman to cycle to anxiety or irritability in a heartbeat. Many women don't know what is happening to them if a normally upbeat personality becomes depressed or moody. The nutritional supplement, SAM-e, is a natural mood enhancer, and very helpful for the symptom of daytime depression. Don't worry though, if moodiness, depression, anxiety, and irritability weren't part of your personality before perimenopause, they probably won't be after perimenopause.

Constant Fatigue – When a woman crawls into bed and sleeps for hours on end, and still feels tired when she gets up, she is most likely well into perimenopause. Nutritional supplements help with this problem.

Mental Vagueness – The wife sat down at the computer and wrote for an hour, and then took a break for lunch. By the time she returned to her computer, she had no idea what she had written, and had to reread everything from just a couple of hours beforehand.

The wife had never experienced memory loss before. Her dad used to say about her, "That girl has a mind like a steel trap."

Indeed, she had to look away from the license plates on the cars and trucks in front of her on the road, or she would memorize all of them inadvertently! One time, a colleague of her husband's left his car with the valet at the hotel. The next day he couldn't find his valet ticket, and felt discombobulated. The wife piped up with the license plate number. Since she had followed him from the airport in their rental car, his license plate number was neatly stowed away with all the other useless license plate numbers in her brain!

Today, as part of her regular nutritional supplement routine, the wife takes Gingko Biloba. It proved instrumental in helping her to maintain her mental acuity.

Insomnia – A wonderful and magical pill called calcium-magnesium-zinc calms most people enough to sleep. It's good for us too. The calcium maintains strong and healthy bones, and is essential for heart health. The magnesium helps with the absorption of calcium, aids with heart health, and helps muscles to relax and avoid stiffness. The zinc supports the immune system, decreases stress levels, and aids with energy metabolism.

Heart Palpitations – If your heart races and you feel short of breath, you might think that you're having a heart attack. The calcium-magnesium-zinc helps with this malady too. The magnesium stabilizes heart rhythm.

Prickly and Tingling Skin – Occasionally, while the wife worked on her computer, the hairs on the tops of her forearms stood up due to the tingling skin. It occurred regularly while the wife was in perimenopause, but disappeared after menopause.

What Are the Symptoms of Menopause?

A sense of loss overwhelms many women. It might feel as if life is over, and that it is time to lie down and die. Unfortunately, we often have other problems associated with the time of life when menopause occurs, such as aging parents, who need more care. When children start to have grandchildren, we automatically move to the slot called the "older generation." These factors can cause depression. Supplementation with SAM-e and melatonin significantly reduces depression.

Surviving the Evolution from Perimenopause to Postmenopause

Management of Perimenopause – The method you choose to manage the discomforts of perimenopause will depend completely on you, and the sets of problems presented in your individual case. Should you take antidepressant drugs or choose natural mood-enhancing supplementation? It's a personal decision. Should you choose hormone replacement therapy or phytoestrogen supplementation, such as soy? That might depend on your medical history.

The wife had a medical history of cancer, and so the doctors guided her away from hormone replacement therapy. Instead, she took the soy each day. One day, she realized that she wasn't taking the full dose suggested on the bottle. When she increased the amount to the full dosage, all of her joint pain miraculously disappeared, too.

Menopause and Osteoporosis – After menopause, women need an increased intake of calcium, preferably with Vitamin D, to build bone density. Women who don't supplement with calcium face a higher risk of fractures.

Proactive Mindset

This time of life demands a proactive point of view. Search diligently for the solutions that will help you through the highs and lows of perimenopause, and don't give up until you find them. You deserve a quality life with hope for the future.

Andropause

12

Anecdote

The man approached his sixtieth birthday, and the woman wanted to do something special for him that he would remember. She informed him cheerily, "Honey, I've saved ten thousand dollars to take you on a trip to Scotland. When can you fit it into your schedule?"

"I don't want to go to Scotland," he replied grumpily, and looked away from her.

"You wouldn't like to go and see the town where your grandfather used to live?" The woman inquired with encouragement. She raised her eyebrows in question.

"No," he responded glumly and closed the topic. The woman felt quite disappointed because she thought that he would enjoy it so much, and it would be a special way in which to commemorate his sixtieth birthday.

"Are you sure?" She asked tentatively, and tilted her head at him.

"I'm positive," he answered a little too quickly.

She frowned at him, and then politely asked, "Is there somewhere else that you'd like to go?"

"No," he said sullenly and shook his head at her. She let it go. He acted so irritable lately that the woman couldn't figure out what was wrong with him.

She sulked away from him and felt sad. "Okay," she said quietly to herself.

On the day of his sixtieth birthday, she draped herself across his lap as he sat in his easy chair, and kissed him passionately. "Would you like to go upstairs? I'll rub your feet for you," she offered and wiggled her eyebrows with humor at him.

"No," he replied, "I'm watching the baseball game." He grimaced at her because she was in his line of vision.

"Oh," she answered with disappointment. She removed herself from his lap and mentioned, "I've made a reservation for dinner tonight at your favorite restaurant."

"Have fun," he retorted unkindly.

Her dander started to rise at his uncooperative attitude and moodiness, "So what are you going to do, sit in the dark all afternoon and evening and feel sorry for yourself?"

"Yep," he rejoined morosely.

"You big poop!" She hollered at him, and gathered a little more steam, "I'm going to the movies without you, and then out to dinner afterwards, so there! Sit in the dark and sulk!" She stomped off without hearing his answer.

"I will," he countered under his breath.

∞

Ten years passed, and now the man's seventieth birthday was closing in on them quickly. The woman remembered his surliness on his sixtieth birthday, and wondered if he'd throw another fit for his seventieth birthday.

She hesitated, and then began, "Your birthday is in two weeks. Would you like to have a little party?"

"No!" he barked at her for no reason at all. She thought that perhaps she should leave him alone before he had another snit. "Besides, I won't be here. I'll be in Bangkok on business."

"I suppose you're not going to tell any of your colleagues that it's your birthday either," she presumed as she eyed him warily.

"That's right," he rejoined rapidly and glared at her.

"Thank God that you'll be gone. I won't have to deal with your childish temper tantrums again for a few more years," the woman chuckled and smiled at him, as they both remembered his sixtieth birthday.

He grimaced at her, and responded, "Good, I'd just like to forget about birthdays from this moment on."

"Fine, but that doesn't let you off the hook for my birthdays! Do you understand?" She snapped at him.

"I've got it!" he growled and left the room.

"Hoh!" she exclaimed, "I'd just like to let him have it!" She smacked her fist in her other hand with exasperation.

What Is Andropause?

Androgens – There are several adrenal androgens, but the primary androgen is testosterone. Mainly, the testicles produce this hormone. That is why researchers refer to male menopause as andropause. To use the term menopause would be a misnomer because the man's testosterone levels do not cease completely like the hormone levels in a woman. Instead, they decline about ten percent every ten years starting around the age of twenty-five. It's different for every man. Some men still have enough testosterone to procreate well into their eighties.

Decline in Testosterone – A man experiences a decline in the production of testosterone as he ages. This could cause him problems as early as the age of forty-five, but markedly after the age of seventy. Researchers claim that low testosterone levels will eventually affect every man. No man escapes the malady if he lives long enough.

What Are the Symptoms of Andropause?

Testosterone Defines Masculinity – When a male becomes a teenager, the testosterone is the hormone, which defines his masculinity. Broader shoulders, a voice change, the growth of a beard, sexual libido, and confident aggression are the characteristics that testosterone creates, a sense of manliness.

Decrease in Manliness Characteristics – Low testosterone decreases the thickness of the beard, and causes the hair on the head to fall out, or to become thinner. When a man was a teenager, the shoulders broadened, and muscle mass increased. With low testosterone, the muscle mass declines as much as ten percent every ten years. Belly fat accumulates around the man's mid-section. Bone loss or osteoporosis begins later than with a woman, but it does occur in an older man's life.

Decrease in Confident Aggression – Testosterone moved a young man to go out into the world and accomplish his goals. Low testosterone can cause depression, a loss in confidence, indecisiveness, forgetfulness, and a sense of having passed one's prime. It might further aggravate a man's life with mood fluctuations, unexpected emotional upset, and a general lack of motivation to achieve.

Decreased Sexual Libido – Many a woman can describe the problems that accompany low testosterone levels. A man experiences fewer early morning erections. His desire and ability to perform sex with his partner decline. Emotionally, he still might love his partner deeply, but his ability to express that love declines sexually. As you know, many medications exist to aid with this problem from Cialis to Viagra. The orgasms of the man decrease in intensity. The man might create a problem in his relationship with his partner to avoid facing the issue of sexual impotency. A man might desire a younger or different partner, and conjure fantasies about such a relationship.

Decline in General Health – Low testosterone can cause joint and muscle pain, upper and lower back pain, hot flashes and flushes or profuse sweating, trouble with going to sleep and staying asleep, constant fatigue, and a loss of fitness. If you feel tired all the time and have no sense of vitality for life, or you have less endurance for physical activity, you might have low testosterone.

Subjective Feelings that Something Is Not Right – The vigor of youth disappears. Low testosterone can cause a loss of interest in leisure-time activities, a sense that one isn't getting anything done, a failure to focus mentally, and a lack of confidence in achievement. A person might withdraw from the world socially, and harbor feelings of anger about life being over, or the person might feel lonely, unattractive, and unloved.

Depression, Anxiety, Nervousness, and Irritability – No one wants anything to do with this four-pack harbinger of doom, but it happens. If life's circumstances set you off easily, or you feel stressed a great portion of the time, the culprit very possibly could be low testosterone.

What Can a Man Do about Andropause?

See Your Doctor – First, find out what is causing the underlying symptoms. The doctor will determine if any other problems exist, which could cause the same symptoms, such as diabetes, prostate cancer, liver or kidney disease, or thyroid problems. Once he has ruled out other maladies, the doctor will order a series of blood tests, which will include the blood testosterone level.

Testosterone Replacement Therapy (TRT) – If the doctor gives you the go ahead to take testosterone replacement therapy, you can look forward to an increased zest for life in the first few weeks, and improved mental acuity. As you continue the therapy, energy and activity will continue to increase, and your interest in sex will return. As several weeks go by, you'll continue to enjoy improving energy and endurance, fat will lessen around the mid-section, and muscle mass will improve.

Mood-Enhancing Supplements or an Antidepressant – The doctor might suggest an antidepressant for the mood swings, or you could try the nutritional supplement SAM-e, which has proven to cure depression in most adults. If your depression is acute, take the full dose.

Melatonin – Melatonin supplementation will take care of any sleeping problems that you have. Surprisingly, the depression might lift as well. Getting a good night's rest is crucial to feeling healthy.

Nutrition – Eat as many vegetables as you can, and cut out refined and processed foods to get rid of belly fat. The nastiest offenders are white bread and pasta. Choose organic foods whenever possible to avoid antibiotics, pesticides, and growth hormones. Take the fat out of your diet, and supplement it with fish oil. Adopt a Mediterranean diet, and use virgin olive oil instead of butter when cooking.

Exercise – You have to expend energy to have energy. Go outside and engage in a physical activity that you enjoy, or develop a regular exercise routine at home, but do something! If you want increased vitality, you need to do the work.

Men Are Sexy Over Fifty

Active men over fifty are the most attractive bunch of men on the planet. The silliness of youth is gone. The trials of raising children are finished, for the most part. The career is established. Now it's time for you to enjoy your life, and make the most out of it. Go forth and conquer the beast who holds you back!

Nutritional Supplements 13

Anecdote

The doctor warned the woman, "Cut out any nutritional supplements and aspirin for two weeks before surgery on your knee."

The woman gazed at the doctor thoughtfully, and wondered what that would do to her energy level, "Okay," she said hesitantly.

He understood her reluctance and reiterated, "This is very important, no nutritional supplements or aspirin for two weeks prior to your surgery." He nodded his head affirmatively and raised his eyebrows for emphasis.

"I understand doctor," the woman replied and sighed.

The next day the woman didn't take any of her supplements, and felt a lack of energy for her workout. She did it anyway, but had to force herself to exercise for the full hour and a half.

While she rode the recumbent bike, the man kissed her on the cheek and said, "I'm on my way to the bank."

"Man, is this ever difficult for me today. I can't imagine how I'm going to feel in two more weeks without supplements!" The woman complained to the man.

"You know what the doctor said," the man reminded her.

"I know," she sighed with disgust.

Two weeks passed by and the day for her surgery approached. The man literally watched his wife turn into an old woman right before his very eyes. She couldn't get herself out of bed at the usual time in the morning. She complained of joint pain, lower back pain, and arthritis in her hands. She acted irritable and depressed, and didn't feel like walking the dogs in the park. She stopped her daily ritual of yard work, and gained three pounds, which caused her to act surlier.

"Thank God that your surgery is tomorrow," the man remarked at her general decline in health.

"Thank God is right. I feel like a witch and something else that rhymes with that word!" She exclaimed with angst.

The man chuckled at her humor, and replied, "You'll feel better soon when you're back on your supplements."

If You Don't Believe in Supplements, You Haven't Tried Them

First Story of Success – Fifteen years ago, after the woman's dad had both his hips replaced, the doctors began to talk to him about having his knees replaced. The hip replacements had gone smoothly, and he was up and active within three weeks. The woman knew that the knees were another story. It takes longer to recuperate from knee replacement. The woman explained to her dad that he should try glucosamine with chondroitin to oil his joints, and she sent him some. He took it every day and became a believer, even though he hadn't supplemented his diet with anything except candy bars for his entire life! He lived another nine years, and never did need the knee replacement surgery.

Second Story of Success – After the woman's knee surgery eight years ago, the surgeon informed her that her knee would only last one or two years, and then it would need replacement. He advised her to continue with the glucosamine with chondroitin, and add the supplement methylsulfonylmethane (MSM). The woman did as the surgeon advised, and her knee still felt strong eight years later without any joint pain or loss of mobility. Her knee worked well enough for her to ski, ride a horse, play golf, work in the yard, ride a bike, and do almost anything within reason.

Regular Supplementation – The wife and her husband took numerous supplements daily. They lined up their little plastic bags about every twenty days, and then filled them with what they needed to stay healthy. They carried the supplement bags with them, wherever they went. Supplementation was a priority for them to keep them out of the doctor's office. They diligently followed this routine for dozens of years. It improved their quality of life, and made growing older a fallacy.

Vitamin Supplementation for Health, Strength, and Energy

The Essentials – Maintain health, strength, and energy with a well-rounded vitamin supplementation plan, which includes nutrients, the omega-3 fatty acids, and the phytonutrients for powerful antioxidant protection. Don't skip on anything. Our bodies need nutrients to stay healthy: Vitamin A, Vitamin C, Vitamin D, Vitamin E, Thiamine, Riboflavin, Niacin, Vitamin B6, Folic Acid, Vitamin B12, Biotin, Pantothenic Acid, Calcium, Magnesium, Zinc, Selenium, Copper, Manganese, Chromium, Molybedenum, Potassium, Choline, Citrus Bioflavonoid Complex, Gamma Tocopherol, Hesperidin, Quercetin, Rutin, Para-aminobenzoic Acid (PABA), Inositol, Alpha Lipoic Acid, Silica, Delta Tocopherol, mixed Tocotrienols, and trace minerals.

Omega -3 Fatty Acids – A fish oil concentrate provides the omega-3 fatty acids we need for immune system and heart health, as well as support for the brain, eyes, and nerves.

Antioxidants – Powerful phytonutrients prevent aging: cinnamon, a blend of fruits, Reserveratol, Lutein, and Lycopene.

Vitamin Packets – Preplanned vitamin packets that contain all the above supplementation are available online and in the stores. Find a complete plan, and stick with it. If you'd like to know which plan we use, just e-mail me. The contact information is at the back of the book.

The Power of Greens

There are many green products to choose from nowadays. Look for a blend that includes vitamins, minerals, grass and bean whole foods, antioxidants, enzymes, and phytonutrients. You'll experience a super-charged energy level from greens. Greens help to lower blood pressure and cholesterol levels, relieve inflammation and stiffness of arthritis, and sharpen mental acuity. They are also beneficial in supporting the immune system, and getting rid of belly fat. Greens will give you beautiful skin and hair. Go green!

Fiber for Weight and Cholesterol Control

Our bodies need 20 to 35 grams of fiber a day. If you are not getting the proper amount of fiber through your diet, then supplement it with Irvingia, in powder form or tablets. Look online for a good source such as LifeExtension. There are several choices on the shelf at your local drugstore too. Fiber is essential to drag the unwanted bile acids and cholesterol out of your body. It also improves sluggish elimination.

Glucosamine with Chondroitin and Methylsulfonylmethane (MSM) for Joint Health

Take the *full* dosage and experience the freedom of feeling younger joints. These two supplements are accumulative, but they will make you feel better within a few days.

Curcumin for Arthritis, High Cholesterol, and Prevention of Cancer

Curcumin, used to make the spice Turmeric and curries, has strong medicinal abilities to help in many areas. It reduces the pain and inflammation of arthritis. It lowers bad cholesterol (LDL) and triglycerides, and raises good cholesterol (HDL). Curcumin is a powerful antioxidant, which can help prevent cancer. Researchers are studying the effects of Curcumin on the prevention of Alzheimer's disease. That would be great news for all of us aging baby boomers.

Gingko Biloba for Memory

If you have trouble remembering where you parked your car at the grocery store, the name of your favorite movie, or what you ate for dinner last night, you will love Gingko Biloba. Get the fuzz out of your brain, and focus on improved memory function by taking Gingko Biloba.

Milk Thistle for Cleansing of the Liver

The liver is the largest organ in our bodies, and we need it to detoxify our bodies. Not only does milk thistle cleanse the liver from toxins, such as alcohol, but it also has restorative abilities to repair liver damage. Used over time, milk thistle can help to regenerate a damaged liver.

SAM-e for Mood Enhancement, Energy, Joints, Liver, and Longevity

Cures Depression in Most Adults – If your depression is acute, take the full dose daily, and encounter the new life before you.

Relieves Depression – The methyl compounds support healthy brain function. No one wants to feel depressed. SAM-e will help you to feel like your old self again.

Boosts Energy Levels – SAM-e helps maximize a workout, and give a person a quick recovery when it is over.

Keeps Connective Tissue Healthy – SAM-e metabolizes glucosamine and chondroitin sulfates, which ensures that cartilage, ligaments, and tendons stay healthy.

Liver Detoxification – SAM-e supports the liver's ability to rid our bodies of free radicals. The metabolism of SAM-e supports the components in the liver needed for detoxification reactions.

Probiotics and Digestive Enzymes for Digestion and Intestinal Health

Degeneration of Probiotics – Probiotics lose their effectiveness rapidly. Leave them in the foil container until you're ready to pop one into your mouth. You want the good bacteria to make it into your intestinal tract.

Digest Dairy Products – If you're lactose intolerant, the taking of the probiotic and the digestive enzyme might solve the problem, and you'll be able to eat dairy products.

Digest Carbohydrates – Eating a high fiber diet means adding more raw fruits and vegetables to your diet, which might cause intestinal gas and bloating. The probiotic and digestive enzyme will take care of that problem too.

Combat Antibiotics – If you have taken an antibiotic recently, replenish the good bacteria in your intestinal tract with a probiotic.

Toxins – The good bacteria in the probiotic neutralize toxins found in the gut.

Increases Absorption of Compounds – Probiotics and digestive enzymes boost the absorption of calcium, magnesium, copper, and iron.

Elimination – Probiotics support regular elimination.

Flax Seed Oil for Overall Health

Irregularity – Adding flax seed oil to your diet will help with irregularity, but it has many other benefits too.

Omega-3 Fatty Acids – It is nature's most bioavailable source of omega-3 fatty acids, which support cardiovascular, circulatory, immune system, nervous system, and joint health.

Colon and Breast Cancer – Researchers have proven that the incidence of colon and breast cancer are significantly lower in people who take flax seed oil.

LDL and Triglycerides – It also helps to lower bad cholesterol and triglyceride levels in the blood.

Numerous Benefits – There are at least twenty more benefits from weight loss to asthma.

Irvingia for Weight Loss, High Cholesterol, and Blood Glucose Levels

Irvingia is a derivative developed from the dika nuts of wild mango, African mango, or bush mango trees. This high-fiber nut is composed of fourteen percent fiber, which might be the reason that it works for weight loss, lowering bad cholesterol, raising good cholesterol, and lowering blood glucose levels. Test groups lost weight and lowered their body fat significantly. Irvingia is new to the health food industry, and therefore, research and studies continue.

Calcium-Magnesium-Zinc for Good Sleep, Calming Nerves, and Wellness

Sleep – Instead of taking a sleeping pill, try calcium-magnesium-zinc tablets to help you sleep at night. They are very effective, and good for you. The zinc supports the immune system, and calcium and magnesium support healthy bones and teeth, and the cardio-vascular system.

Calms Nerves – Take a calcium-magnesium-zinc one hour before any speech, presentation, or performance, and any nerves will disappear.

Green Tea Extract for Staying Cancer Free

An Antioxidant – Green tea is an antioxidant that is twenty times more active than Vitamin C. That is an amazing truth.

An Anticarcinogenic – It is a powerful anticarcinogenic that inhibits cancer cells. Components in green tea extract actually block the growth of cancer cells, and promote the death of them.

An Anti-inflammatory – Green tea extract has proven to treat chronic inflammation successfully.

Coenzyme Q10 for Cell Function

The body manufactures Coenzyme Q10 for the proper functioning of cells. As we grow older, Coenzyme Q10 levels often decrease. Research has reported that people with chronic diseases, such as heart conditions, diabetes, cancer, etc., also have lower levels of Coenzyme Q10. We can increase the amount of Coenzyme Q10 in our bodies through supplementation if our bodies are not producing enough of it. However, Coenzyme Q10 remains highly controversial as a treatment for high blood pressure, macular degeneration, asthma, cancer, heart health, and a number of other health issues.

Acetyl L- Carnitine for Mental Acuity

Acetyl L-Carnitine aids people with mental vagueness and fatigue, lack of motivation, and mild depression, and helps with diseases that cause these symptoms. Red meat is an excellent source of Acetyl L-Carnitine. If you don't eat red meat, and notice that you have not been feeling mentally sharp, it's possible that Acetyl L-Carnitine supplementation could help you.

Soy Isoflavones for Men and Women for Prevention of Cancer and Much More

Food Source – Soy isoflavones are in the food source of soybeans.

Calm Perimenopause Symptoms – Supplementation with soy lessens perimenopause symptoms, primarily the hot flashes.

Prevent Enlargement of the Prostate – Men should also take soy to help prevent enlargement of the prostate gland.

Prevent Breast, Endometrial, and Prostate Cancer – It is also a powerful substance to help defeat cancer by causing the cancer cells to die. It has proven to protect from breast, endometrial, and prostate cancer. It is so effective in protection from tumors that it actually acts similar to drugs used to treat cancer.

Reduce Heart Disease – Soy isoflavones reduce the risk of heart disease by inhibiting the growth of plaque that clogs arteries, and it reduces cholesterol.

Build Bones – Soy helps prevent osteoporosis by preserving the bones. Many studies also suggest that it increases bone density in women.

Relief from Joint and Back Pain – One day while the wife watched television, an Indian doctor explained the benefits of soy to joint and back pain. She had never heard that before, and so she checked the recommended dosage on the bottle of soy isoflavones. She found that she was only taking one-fourth of the recommended dosage. When she increased her dosage to the full amount, every lingering bit of joint and lower back pain disappeared.

Relief from Arthritis – New studies suggest that soy isoflavones might relieve arthritis in men.

L-Arginine for Prevention of Heart Disease and Erectile Dysfunction

L-Arginine, produced mainly in the kidneys and to a lesser extent in the liver, is an essential amino acid for the body. Supplementation might not be necessary, unless your source of L-Arginine was depleted due to an injury or infection. L-Arginine helps to relax blood vessels, increases the flow of blood, and supports the functioning of blood vessels. Therefore, it might be helpful for people with heart disease, erectile dysfunction, high blood pressure, or vascular claudication.

Niacin for Men for the Enjoyment of Sex

Niacin expands the small capillaries to allow the flow of more blood cells. Although it is necessary for many functions in the body, it is essential in the synthesis of testosterone. Niacin supplementation can increase a man's sexual potency, and enhance his orgasms. After taking the niacin, men report a flush, which warms the skin and causes it to tingle. The flush is harmless if you don't mind the sensation.

Dehydroepiandrosterone (DHEA) for Aging

The vote is still out on DHEA. As we grow older, the DHEA levels in our bodies decrease, which means that lean muscle mass and bone density decline, and the immune system sags. Some people swear by DHEA, but the studies don't support their interest in it. The Mayo Clinic conducted a two-year study, which resulted in no significant changes. We need more research for definitive support of DHEA. However, if you don't want to wait for conclusive research, take it to hedge your bets.

Nutrition for the Skin

Miraculous Renewal – The nail specialist was finishing the wife's nails when a representative arrived at the salon to make a presentation to him. The man showed the nail specialist and the wife a galvanic spa made by Nu Skin, and told them that it rejuvenated the skin. The wife didn't know if the manicurist was interested, but she was, anything to help with aging skin. The man showed her the hand held device, and how it worked. She had heard about it, but had never used it. The man gave her a treatment on the right side of her face. The results were astonishing! When she looked in the mirror, the right side of her face appeared plumped, fresh, and youthful, and most of the fine wrinkles were gone, along with the puffiness under her eyes. The left side of her face looked like a sad sister in comparison! With such dramatic results, the wife bought the Nu Skin Galvanic Spa.

Experimenting with the Device – The wife began experimenting with the device and the two to five minute treatments, and discovered many interesting things. When she used it on her sagging inner thighs, they plumped and firmed up, and the cellulite disappeared. When she used it on her belly, her jeans grew looser as the belly fat diminished. When she used the instrument underneath her arms, the skin stopped sagging. When she used it on her décolleté, all the fine wrinkles disappeared, and the skin appeared smooth and lovely.

One day the wife bumped against a flowerpot, and a nasty bruise appeared on her knee. She didn't know if the device would help or not, but she thought she'd try it. For three days in a row, she massaged the bruise with the galvanic spa, and on the fourth day, the bruise was gone. Usually, her bruises took eight to ten days to discolor.

Current Routine – With ecstatic delight in the results, the wife established a regular routine. On Mondays, she treated her upper thighs.

On Tuesdays, she treated her arms, the whole arm, and not just the sagging under arm. The reason was that it changed the texture of the skin by delivering vital nutrients to the skin. The result was a smooth and much younger appearing epidermis.

On Wednesdays, the wife worked on her face and décolleté. On Thursdays, she worked on her belly, and her upper thighs. On Fridays, she worked on her arms and her belly. On Saturdays, she worked on her face and décolleté again. The wife took Sunday off.

Public Declarations – People began complimenting the wife on her skin everywhere she went, and asked her what her beauty secret was.

Most people have heard about the Nu Skin Galvanic Spa, but haven't tried it, or don't want to get involved in a business. The truth is that you can just buy the amazing instrument, and you don't have to do the business. If you decide you want to be a distributor, you can simply sign up later. If you'd like to know how to purchase the Galvanic Spa, just e-mail me at –

sexyatsixty@live.com

and I'll input your information so that you can go online and place whatever orders that you like. Soon you'll be the envy of all your friends, and feel much better about living in your second half.

Spirituality

Anecdote

The wife was a member of the one-hundred-forty voice choir at church. The choir performed a musical for the congregation before taking the summer off. The husband sat up high in the pitched section of the large sanctuary, and waited for the production to begin. The famous choir director conducted a thirty-eight piece orchestra. He cued them to begin the introduction. The doors of the sanctuary flew open and the massive choir marched down the aisles singing.

Thrilling shouts of joy and excitement reverberated throughout the large auditorium, as the congregation stood, cheered, and clapped their hands. The husband watched from the back of the auditorium and a lump formed in his throat. The famous choir director knew how to reach into the hearts of the audience and touch them.

The choir members marched up onto the bleachers, and continued to clap their hands with the audience. The famous director directed the orchestra and the choir at the same time, an amazing feat unequaled by another director in their church, but then he was a professional. The song ended, and the congregation gave a rousing standing ovation to the choir and orchestra.

The director cued the orchestra to begin the next number, and the choir tenderly sang the words of the verse. Timpani drums pumped the song with new energy, and the choir erupted into four-part harmony for the chorus. A fellow choir member, who was late in arriving at church, hustled out onto the stage and pushed her way up onto the third bleacher step. The row of singers shuffled each other to the end of the row to make room, and the wife, who stood on the end, fell off the bleacher to the floor! Her husband, watching the debacle from the back of the giant sanctuary, covered his mouth with embarrassment.

The choir sang, "You're my sister. You're my brother. Take my hand."

The man standing next to the wife, who now stood down on the floor of the stage, reached his hand down to the wife and hauled her up onto the bleacher, and then steadied her on the end. The woman next to him grabbed his hand to steady him, and the remainder of the choir followed suit. Everyone joined hands, and moved as one from right to left as they shifted their weight from foot to foot in the rousing version of the song.

"You're my sister. You're my brother. Take my hand," they sang with uplifting enthusiasm.

People in the congregation stood as the words of the song filled their hearts with exultation. They joined hands, and reached across the aisles to the members on the other side. The people on the end of each long row subdivided and grabbed the hand of the person at the end of the next row until the entire congregation of two-thousand-eight-hundred people connected and moved back and forth as one with the choir.

Tears sprang up in the eyes of the husband as he said to his friend,

"Jesus is marching in the aisles."

The choir watched in amazement from the stage as the whole of the sisters and brothers in Christ in the large hall proclaimed together, "You're my sister. You're my brother. Take my hand."

The famous choir director glanced over his shoulder at the audience, and tears of gratefulness clouded his eyes, as the message of the song reached inside the hearts of everyone present and drove the point home.

"Thank you Father," he said as he looked up at his Maker.

The husband's friend said to the husband, "I can see why your wife likes choir so much."

The husband nodded in agreement, and then reached for his hanky to blow his nose. He replied with a catch in his throat, "God's hand moves across the planet."

Average Time Spent Worshiping

The Ladies Home Journal published an interesting analysis about how the average person spent his or her time. The article revealed the following: six years are spent in eating; eleven years in working; five and a half years in washing and dressing; three years in education; eight years in amusement; six years in walking; three years in reading; three years in conversation; twenty-four years in sleeping, and just six months in worshiping God.

The Way We Were Made

God made our eyes to look ahead. He made our nose to point forward, and planted the mouth conveniently just below the nose, in front of us where we could reach it. Our feet walk forward, and our arms face forward. Do you think that maybe God wanted us to go forward? If you are fifty or over, chances are you have already lived more than half of your life. What are you marching towards,

Heaven? There isn't that much time left to get this part of your life right. Perhaps it's time to connect with the Source, if you haven't already done so.

You Can't Save Yourself

Personal Power Versus God's Power – Jesus did not come to earth to encourage us to save ourselves from sin. His Father sent him to earth to do it for us, because God knew we couldn't do it for ourselves. Some people believe that their accomplishments come from the power that exists within them. They feel that they have an internal ability to act in a right manner. They believe that it is innate. They claim to be good people, and an outward examination reveals that they are indeed admirable people. An inward examination exposes the faultiness of those beliefs. How can a person live an entire life, and believe that they have not once had a sinful thought, word, or action? Maybe the person believes that a little sin is okay. However, God is blameless. To be acceptable to him, we must also be blameless. We no more have the power to save ourselves from sin than we would have the power to raise ourselves from the dead.

Born without Sin – The virgin birth is very important because Jesus could not have the sinful nature of Adam, like all other blemished human beings. The Son of God had to be born without any sin. He was born of a woman, Mary, and yet, he was fully human, *and* he is completely divine. Because he is God, he has the power to deliver us from our sins because he has the power to overcome death.

Humans All Sin – When we are born again, the Holy Spirit comes to reside within us. The Holy Spirit blesses us with his teaching, but also convicts us of our evil thoughts and deeds. The giant mountain of coal piled on our heads becomes readily apparent, and we understand that we cannot save ourselves from our sin. We purposefully turn from our sinful nature, but we are never able to be one-hundred percent without sin. When a human being believes that he or she has the power within to save his own person from sin, the person, in a sense, believes that he or she is his or her own god, but there is only one God.

Supernatural Birth – Jesus' virgin birth was supernatural. For anyone to believe that a virgin birth was possible, the person would have to believe in God. Perhaps that is why there are so many cynics because sometimes it's just simpler not to believe. The two most significant events of all time are Jesus' virgin birth, and his taking of all our sins on the cross and rising from the dead.

Temptations – As a human being, Jesus had temptations, just as we all have temptations. However, he did not sin, but instead, was holy and blameless. He understood our struggles, and he knew that we could not save ourselves from our human condition of sin. We can try as hard as we like, but it will never happen. It is like the anecdote about Benjamin Franklin. He made a list of all the character traits that he would like to have, and then he set out to manifest those traits in himself. When he completed working through his list, he announced his success in achieving the traits, but added that he now lacked humility! Our human condition is similar to that. Even though we may be good, we will never be perfect like God. Only Jesus can save us from our sins.

We Were All Created to Worship

Desire to Worship – Everyone can see that this is true if you look at all the things and people, who we worship. Hero worship is everywhere. People worship sports stars, movie stars, rock stars, racecar stars, athletic stars, dancing stars, soap opera stars, motivational stars, political stars, and stars in every occupation. Some people worship things like jewelry, cars, houses, and collector items. Others worship places, such as mountains, beaches, and parks. Some people worship money and credit cards. What does that tell you about us? It tells you that we have a need to look up to someone or something, an innate, built-in need to worship. We all have a desire to worship. The Lord gives us a solid reason to worship him.

Manmade God – All the above things that we worship are idols. Anything that we give power or value to is an idol, a manmade god. The manmade god might provide immediate gratification, but nothing that is lasting. The manmade god did not create us. We cannot trust a manmade god. A manmade god does not give us God's truth. The manmade god does not give us a reason to live for eternity. A manmade god does not forgive our sins.

Privilege to Worship God Directly – When Jesus came to earth, died for us, and rose again, he changed the old order of things. We no longer have to go through someone else to worship. We have the privilege of worshiping our Lord directly. God is everywhere all the time. We can worship him anytime: walking, sitting, riding in a car, eating in a restaurant, lying down, in a plane, on a beach, or riding in a chairlift. He welcomes all our worship.

Worship Changes Who We Are – When we worship, the Holy Spirit goes to work to change us. The act of worship gives our spirit a chance to commune with God. No one is the same after spending time with God. The Holy Spirit asks the Lord for the exact right thing that we need, even when we are not aware of what that might be. It might be the realization that we are not first, and it is not about us. It is all about Jesus. We worship him because of what he has done for us, given us the gift of forgiveness so that we don't have to live continually in sin and guilt.

From Microbe to Man?

Ongoing Time Continuum – The husband took a snapshot of his wife at the beach. It was a perfect moment in time with the late afternoon lighting the gulf waters and the tide rolling in on cue. The snapshot was less than a second of the woman's life, and yet when one viewed it, one could see the coordination of an ongoing time continuum that maintains the light and the dark, and the planets in alignment so that the sun and moon can rise and set, and incoming and outgoing tides could arrive on schedule.

Coordination of Time and the World – If one took that time continuum for one person and stretched it over the space of the person's lifetime, it would seem nothing short of miraculous that all the pieces held together in perfect coordination. If one took the time continuum and stretched it from the beginning of time to the end of time, and then multiplied it by the number of people who have ever lived, and calculated the permutations and combinations, it is impossible to believe that the orchestration of that world happened randomly.

A Superior Power – If one viewed the perfect order in which all those people existed under a predictable moon and sun, among meticulously accurate planets, it would only seem possible that an entity of superior power had conceived of it.

Miracle of the Human Body – Add to the picture, the number of organs and functions in a body, and how they work together so perfectly to maintain the human in a state either of homeostasis or of adapted imbalance. Add the number of critically aligned elements that must operate in coordination to create an ongoing physical history, and the mind cannot conceive of anything that vast and universal.

Overwhelming Evidence – The evidence is too overwhelming to ignore. God lives and watches from way out there in his third heaven. We have unending miracles for which to be thankful, even if we are just standing here and doing nothing. It isn't that hard to believe in God.

Journey to Paradise – Lilia's Story

I wrote the following piece as a prologue for a future book:

Lilia approached the end of her life on earth. She had no one remaining to watch her die. Her mother and father had passed on long ago, and her husband had died a few years earlier. Her breaths labored, but she felt no agony in her spirit. She didn't need to worry about her past anymore. She knew unconsciousness was approaching, but she didn't struggle to stay alert. She would relent to death when the time came.

Lilia knew she had made mistakes, but she no longer had any regrets. She wished that she could go back and fix the many wrongs she had committed that affected others' lives. Lilia also wished that she could return to her beloved Kauai one more time before she died, but that was not to be. The doctors told her she might have a few months. Doctors always said things like that to give the patient hope. Lilia didn't have to worry about hope because she knew that God had built eternity into the heart of man by giving man the desire to live forever.

Lilia knew she wasn't going to live forever, not on this earth. She hoped that she would close her eyes and go into a coma, so that when her breathing slowed, she didn't have to worry about the suddenness of life being over. That is the way it was with her father. He didn't suffer, but simply faded away. Lilia was definitely failing, but she thought to herself, *I'm just going to close my eyes and think about my life.*

Lilia saw the beautiful palm trees, and heard the swishing of their branches in the gentle trade winds. She pictured her island with its lush tropical flowers, trees, and plants growing almost everywhere. She smelled the fragrant seedpods of the mokihana, the flower of Kauai. She imagined the mokihana strung into a lei necklace with some maile leaves, and felt it sitting gently on her skin. She envisioned the Fern Grotto, up the Wailua River, at the mouth of a lava cave. The ferns and philodendrons glistened in the sunshine after a rainfall. Lilia imagined and smelled the wild ginger and hibiscus.

Lilia revisited the place where the banana plants grew wild alongside the road to Poipu. She sat underneath the enormous majestic coconut palms at the Coco Palms Resort, palms that her grandfather had planted many years before. Lilia sat on the veranda of their family home in Wailua. She had loved living in Wailua's rural, down-to-earth atmosphere. She smelled the sugar cane fields burning after a harvest, sweet, tangy, and smoky in the wind. After her death, her sister would throw her ashes into the ocean in Wailua Bay at Lilia's request, and then she would be home forever. Lilia was born in paradise, and she would live in Paradise again soon.

Fashion Mojo

Anecdote

The man and woman traveled to Hawaii for a well-earned vacation. They arrived at the hotel, and quickly dressed in their swimsuits and cover-ups. The man pulled on his new blue swimming trunks with white top stitching, which ended right above his kneecap. He pulled on a matching t-shirt with a convenient pocket on the right side of his chest for his sunglasses.

He slipped on his leather sandals, and announced, "I'm ready."

"You look very stylish dear. What happened to the old swimming trunks?" The woman asked him as she quirked her eyebrow at him. He usually wore things until they fell apart, which meant that she had to endure the embarrassing deterioration of the garment before it found its way into the ragbag.

"I thought you'd like us to look as if we actually go together," he chuckled and grinned, proud of himself.

"Thank you honey, I appreciate that. You'll look great in the pictures I plan to take of you next to our palm tree," she smiled at him wickedly. "You've still got it, you handsome hunk."

"I'm glad that you think so," he replied with an engaging smile.

The woman pulled on a tasteful and shapely one-piece swimsuit, which fit her perfectly, and displayed her curves. The top of the suit sported varying colors of turquoise, which turned to purple beneath the chest, and then black at the waist. She pulled on her black swim pants, sharp enough to wear out for the evening. She slipped her well-manicured toes into high-heeled wedge sandals to improve her walking and standing posture. She added her diamond wedding ring and matching bracelet on her left hand and wrist, and a silver bracelet and topaz ring set in white gold on her right hand and wrist. She pulled her shiny hair back off her face, rolled it up in a colorful turquoise band, and positioned a turquoise cowgirl hat on her head for face protection. She stood to her full height, walked to the closet, and pulled out a long shawl to match her cowgirl hat. She folded it in thirds, and draped it over her shoulder. If they ate in air-conditioning, she would have something to keep her neck and shoulders warm.

The couple proceeded to the beach where they requested two lounge chairs, towels, and an umbrella. Since their plane had not come in until the afternoon, the attendant had no choice but to position them in the third tier of people behind the first two rows that sat closer to the ocean. The woman sighed deeply with pleasure, removed her swim pants and sandals, and reclined gracefully in the lounge chair. The man and woman sat on the sand of the beach at Waikiki and admired the ever-changing blues of the Pacific.

Many beach goers occupied the beach in front of them. Lying on a sand mat directly in front of the man and woman was a tall, but overweight grandma, who appeared to be in her late seventies. Her tan was so dark that her skin appeared muddy and ruddy. She wore a bikini. The top fitted her poorly, and offered little support for her breasts. They drooped down and lied on top of the many folds of her dark brown un-toned stomach. The woman glanced away from the grandma with embarrassment because the folds of flesh around the grandma's middle and on her thighs made it appear as if she wore no bottom to her bikini! The woman knew that the grandma probably wore a bikini bottom, but the mounds of flesh around it hid it from view! The man smirked and shook his head back and forth at the shocked expression on the woman's face.

Sitting next to the grandma was a grandpa with fair skin. He had on worn, tight-fitting white swim trunks, with a thinning liner, which didn't give his legs or anything else adequate coverage. He wore a light long-sleeve shirt with the buttons fastened around his wrists. He had white gloves on his hands and a floppy white hat on his head, which he had tied under his chin. The grandpa and grandma appeared to be around the same age.

The woman speculated that the older couple probably came to the beach every day. Because the grandpa had fair skin, he had to cover it up to protect himself. The woman felt certain that the grandma had been a spectacular beauty in her youth, and still felt that way. *It is nice that the grandma has good self-esteem*, the woman thought and smiled. *I wish I could buy her a different swimsuit, though.*

A young husband and wife, who had just arrived at the beach, broke into laughter and pointed at the grandma. The woman glimpsed down and felt empathetic discomfiture for the grandma. The grandma stood to her full imposing height, shook out her beach mat, and slipped a see-through cover-up over her swimsuit. She grunted with umbrage at the couple that made fun of her, and stomped her feet in the sand.

She snapped at her partner, "I'm going home. Some people are so rude." She slapped her flip-flops through the sand away from him. The grandpa begrudgingly stood, gathered his towel, and followed her.

The woman gazed meaningfully at the man and felt sad for the older couple. She said, "They have just as much right to enjoy the beach as anyone else."

"It's too bad that you can't give the grandma a makeover," he said with concern for the older couple's feelings.

"Actually, I really wish I could. She had such cute hair!" The woman said with sincerity. "The only problem she has is that she got stuck in the wrong decade."

"Apparently so," the man replied.

He returned to his book to end the conversation. He understood the connection that the woman had with other people, and didn't want her to feel forlorn about it for the rest of the afternoon. He glanced up to see the woman staring at the laughing newcomers.

The man grabbed the woman's hand, and pulled her out of the lounge. "Come on, honey, let's go for a swim," he suggested and hoped it would successfully distract her.

Stuck in the Wrong Decade

The husband and wife knew several people who had style in the 1970s, but who never moved forward after that. One of these individuals still wore a beehive hairdo, mini-skirts, and hot boots some forty years later! It was a little shocking when they saw the woman at reunions because she was well into her seventies. The husband and wife understood that the woman felt in her prime back then, and didn't want to lose the magical feeling, and that's why the woman persisted in sustaining the wardrobe from that period. The wife pondered if changing one thing would be enough, and the answer was a definitive "No." The wife speculated that the woman might be able to get away with the boots if her skirts were longer, and covered the sagging inner thighs. *The hairdo definitely dates her though*, thought the wife. *She would appear much younger if she updated her hair. She needs to get a sense of her fashion mojo to regain her credibility.*

Accessorize for Fashion Mojo

Most people over fifty can't wear the same things that young people wear today because the styles would make them look ridiculous. However, you can choose an accessory that would update your appearance, or change it up in your own way. It's fun and exciting to figure out how the next new trend will fit into your life. The updated looks invigorate the way a person feels, and gives the person more confidence.

Dark Wash Jeans

The Shape of the Leg – Every man and woman should have a great-fitting pair of dark wash jeans. This is a necessary staple for your wardrobe. Choose a straight leg, or a leg that is slightly fuller from the lower thigh to the floor. A person has to be extremely fit to wear a pair of tight-fitting, low-rise, boot-cut jeans.

Choices for Men – Men can team the jeans up with a casual jacket or a sports coat for an updated and classy style. Wear a top underneath, which has a finished neckline. Add leather shoes with a polished finish or half boots.

Choices for Women – Women can pair the jeans up with a casual jacket or a jacket from a suit. Be creative. Take a classic Chanel jacket, add a finished top underneath, and wear it with dark wash jeans. It is a sophisticated, and yet updated and chic look. It is much more interesting than wearing a matching pantsuit or jean suit. That's a little too predictable. For a different twist, roll up the hem of the jean, and add a sassy pair of high-heeled shoes, or tuck the jeans into a pair of stylish boots.

Capri Jeans – Forget about Capri jeans, unless you have very long legs. Many short women love to wear Capri jeans because they don't have to hem the pants, but the truth is that Capri jeans make them appear even shorter. Petite women, do your due diligence, and take your jeans to a tailor.

Banish the Little Black Dress

The basic little black dress is a fallback for women who don't want to think about what to wear. It still lurks in the stores, but you're better off without it, unless it has interesting details. You have an opportunity to divulge more of your personality if you give your appearance a little thought, and add a splash of color. Many women wear black to hide extra weight. Black doesn't diminish your size. It only announces that you're endeavoring to camouflage your weight.

Neutrals Don't Have to Be Boring

Forget about pairing beige with beige. You aren't your grandmother or your grandfather. Mix it up. Try rust with black and grey or brown. Look for crisp sharp colors that aren't dull in appearance. If you wear a plaid jacket with a matching skirt or pant, choose a top with a different dynamic, such as broad diagonal stripes. Find individual pieces that have camaraderie with other unrelated pieces. Doing so makes a very versatile wardrobe.

Caps, Hats, and Fedoras

Turned-Up Brims – Newsboy caps, baker boy caps, cabbie caps, and fedoras with a turned-up brim are an easy way to trend your look. Try the caps on for height of the crown and the size of the bill and brim. Scale the cap or hat to the size of your head. If you have a larger head, wear a cap with a higher crown, and a wider brim. Hats that do not have a turned-up brim squash a person's face. If your intention is to look grim, a flat brim will do it.

Floppy-Brimmed Hats – Many women wear wide-brimmed, floppy straw hats to the beach or to a pool. Nothing announces a person's age as much as one of these hats. You can protect your face in a more fashionable manner. Sport a cowgirl hat with a medium shapeable brim. Turn the brim up a little on the sides, and leave the back and front flat for sun protection. Every head will turn next time you arrive at the pool, and soon the other women will copy your style. Sassy!

High-Heeled Shoes

Platform Shoes – If you've already worn a trend when you were younger, don't repeat it. Mature women look as if they're stuck in the past when they try to repeat it. Why would you want to risk breaking an ankle anyway? There are so many shoe choices today that we didn't have thirty or forty years ago. Choose a shoe that is lovely, but more sensible if you have joint pain. Wearing extremely high heels is very hard on the knees.

High Heels versus Wedges – High-heeled shoes have an allure about them. That's fine if you don't have to stand on your feet for hours on end. If you do have to stand for several hours, choose a wedge instead. It doesn't kill the feet or destroy the knees, *and* it feels more stable.

Boots, Baby!

Tall Boots – A sleek pair of tall leather boots looks smart with skirts, dresses, jeans, and slacks. Boots support the ankles, and make a person feel swank. If the boots have details that you don't want to hide, then tuck the pants into the boots. A draping jersey pant tucked into a trendy boot makes the boot the center of attention.

Half Boots – Let the younger generation wear the platform half boots. They only look good with a shorter skirt so that the leg doesn't lose its proportion.

Over-the-Knee Boots – Unless you're going out on tour with a band, don't wear these boots. You'd have to wear a mid-thigh skirt to prevent the leg from appearing out of proportion.

Black Leather Pants

Black leather jeans or pants look fantastic on slender and tall women or men. If you aren't lithe and sleek, it will only make you look like you're trying to be something that you are not. Women can pair the black leather jeans with a special sweater and high-heeled boots. Men can pair the jeans with a sweater or a sports coat, and polished half boots.

Belts and Waistlines

Women – Are you the narrowest at your waistline, just below your waistline, or below your chest? If you choose to wear a belt, wear it at the smallest point.

Men – A belt looks at its best just below your natural waistline, and not at the top of your thighs. Women will look away if they see too much of your underwear, a butt crack, or think that you're about to lose your pants. Walking around with one hand on your pants to hold them up is just plain unattractive!

The Perfect Leather Jacket

Women – It can be almost any color from turquoise to bright red to basic black with interesting adornments. It is just as easy to coordinate an outfit to go with the turquoise jacket, as it is the black jacket. Scale the length of the jacket to your height, and ensure that it has darts, which tailor the jacket to your waistline. A boxy jacket doesn't flatter many women, no matter your size.

Men – You have many choices from a casual leather bomber jacket to a tailored, leather sport coat. Scale the jacket to your height and size. An oversized jacket on a short man with a slight frame looks like the man is attempting to compensate for his size. You don't' want to appear insecure. Women are attracted to men who have a reasonable sense of their own worth.

The Midriff and Cleavage

Exception – Unless you are at the beach, don't display too much cleavage or your midriff, even if you sport a defined six-pack of abs.

The Midriff – The display of too much skin sends a message about your character. Most people over fifty wouldn't do this anyway, but I've seen a few at the grocery store. Their sagging middles stop traffic they look so inappropriate.

Cleavage – The display of too much cleavage on a mature woman is not sexy. If the skin doesn't fit tight, and the mounds aren't perky anymore, keep them under decent cover. A jelly-like bouncing of the breasts only reveals a loss of elasticity. No one needs to know that except your partner.

Outrageous Trends

When I owned a clothing store, we traveled to the fashion mart every three months for a buying trip. The big marts had a fashion show that filled an auditorium with people. Some of the styles were completely outrageous, but they made the fashion show more fun. That is where outlandish trends belong, on the runway. I can't think of anywhere else a person would wear them. Even if you wore them to the Academy Awards, the press would label you as the worst dressed person attending.

Argyle Leggings and Fishnet Stockings

These are dashing on a young woman with long legs wearing clothing that doesn't compete with the pattern of the leggings or stocking. When we see a young woman or movie star pull this off, we admire them because it isn't easy to do. The rest of us should let them have the fun.

See-Through Clothing

Wear a lovely see-through blouse with a beautiful camisole underneath it. The viewer will notice the shape of your shoulders and shoulder blades, which are slender on almost everyone.

The Duster

It's sexy on both men and women. For this choice of fashion to work, the style must be simple, without embellishment, and no longer than mid-calf.

Bright Red Lipstick and Lip Gloss

Fashion magazines claim that anyone can wear brilliant red lipstick, but if you have white hair or wrinkled skin, it is a mistake. It is too harsh in appearance. If red is your favorite color, choose a softer shade of red, and let it complement your skin tones and eyes.

Necklaces

Chunky Necklaces – They are super-hip right now, but be careful. Heavy jewelry, if worn every day, will create tags on your neck. Save the chunky necklace for a special occasion.

Waist-length Necklaces – At this age, we don't want anything to drag us down, not long hair worn down, and not a necklace worn to the waist. The necklace acts like an arrow and points right at a person's belly. Most people don't want their belly to be the focus of attention.

Proportion – Ensure that necklaces are in proportion to your size. A super-chunky necklace on a petite frame is overwhelming.

Cleavage Necklaces – A necklace that hangs down to your cleavage is a cleavage necklace. They are lovely and quite becoming on most people if the end of the necklace doesn't lodge in between the mounds. A cleavage necklace also needs to be in proportion with your size.

The Wrinkled Rich

In the old movies, the male lead often wore a linen suit that was sloppy and unkempt. The wrinkled look sent the message that the man was rich because he could afford to wear linen. Designers will never move completely away from a sloppy look entirely because it makes some people feel like he or she is the cool cat. When a person has lived fifty years, the only thing we want to see slipshod is a tailored shirt worn with the tails out over a pair of sharp jeans.

Mascara and Makeup

The trend is to wear mascara that is thick and full, the fuller the better. Makeup that appears natural on your face complements a person's features. Makeup that is outrageously thick or over done is clownish. When eyelashes look like a humming bird in flight, there is too much. When a foundation ends suddenly by the ear, it is mask-like in appearance. Keep makeup as natural as possible.

Bone Structure and Design

Large Patterns – Large-boned men and women can wear bolder patterns. The rule of thumb is to relate the pattern to the size of your bone structure. A large pattern worn on a petite person dwarfs him or her.

Proportion – If you have a larger frame, wear clothing that fits you. If you cloak yourself in oversized clothing, you'll lose your shape.

Shoes and Purse Don't Have to Match

Nowadays, the shoes and the purse are accessories, which give us clues about your personality. A pop of color is interesting and confident looking. They don't have to match, but they do have to complement each other.

Wide Horizontal Stripes

If you wear a pencil thin skirt, which looks fabulous on you, and you'd like to make it the focus of attention, wear a wide horizontal stripe on top. Any other time, the wide stripe only adds breadth to the person.

Skin Tight Pants

Reserve them for lithe young people and rock stars, especially if you have to lie down on the floor to get them zipped! Pants should fit your form, and not squeeze you into a sausage.

Long Hair

Older people don't look good with long hair hanging down on either side of their face. It drags the face down. If you have long hair, and like to wear it down, style it to move away from your face so that the focus remains on the face, and not on your hair.

Don't Over-Accessorize

Keep it simple. You don't need outrageous boots with many details paired with a flowered skirt, and then topped with a blouse with a necktie, a necklace, a scarf, and a cape. That's too much. What do you want the viewer to focus on? Most people want the viewer to focus on their face. Less is more.

Search for a Simpler Life

Anecdote

The woman prepared to go to Hawaii. She pulled out the turquoise tops and white shorts and jeans, and laid them out on the oversized chair and ottoman. She laid out her white shoes, all three styles, and pondered if she would need all three. She decided to wear the full casual shoes with her white jeans on the airplane, and set them aside with a white sailor jacket. She hung the second sailor jacket on the bathroom door to pack.

She scuttled downstairs, and opened the closet door where her Newsboy caps hung on hooks ready for any occasion. She picked out three, and then trotted back upstairs. She scrambled to the far end of her first closet, pulled out her cowgirl hats, and another bin full of Newsboy caps, and chose seven hats to match the outfits that she had laid out in both bedrooms. She set one cap aside to wear on the airplane.

She had six bathing suits in three different styles of black, and turquoise. She laid them all out, and the three pairs of black, full-length swim pants that she wore over them. The swim pants looked so good on her that she often wore them out to dinner with a special top. The man had told her to bring something nice because he was going to take her dancing to her favorite spot high above Waikiki Beach. She hustled back to the closet, and pulled out three knit sleeveless and sexy black tops to go with the swim pants. She hooked the hangers on the door to the bedroom, and then returned to the closet to find scarves or shawls to match each one.

Before she forgot her swim sandals, she hurried back into the bathroom, and chose three pairs, a black pair, a turquoise pair, and a beige pair. She grabbed all three and lined them up on top of the dog kennels.

She looked through her second closet, and spied the red jacket and several red tops. She surmised that they would go well with her swim pants too. The dress slacks hung right next to the red tops and jacket in the closet. She pulled out two pairs of black dress slacks, the red tops, and laid them out on the guest bed. She hustled to the second closet, found scarves to match, and added those to the red tops and dress slacks.

The woman opened her third chest of drawers, and perused through the sandals. She had three sets of strappy sandals in black and silver in three distinct styles. She lined the shoes up on top of the dog kennel with the other shoes, and contemplated which shoes would serve her vacation needs the best.

At the back of her third closet, she found the beautiful negligee and bathrobe that she had sewn for herself years ago. She slipped it on, and found that it fit her perfectly. She laid that out on the bed. The negligee made her think of a sexy black short nightgown that resided in her second chest of drawers. She dug through the drawer until she found it. It sat neatly folded right next to several lacy black camisoles.

"I forgot that I even had these," she commented to herself, and pulled out two of the camisoles for the trip.

"Maybe a skirt or two would be nice," she smiled to herself.

She rummaged under the guest bed in the guest bedroom, and pulled out a flat plastic container filled with skirts. She opened it up, and looked through all the skirts. She chose two skirts and two tube tops. She removed them from the container, and shoved it back under the bed. She glanced at the second plastic container under the bed, and yanked it out. Two pairs of very spiffy boots, black and brown, caught her eye. She removed them and pulled out the gaucho pants and matching tops that went with them.

"Maybe I'll wear this on the plane instead," she mused to herself.

The man sat in the living room and watched the baseball game while he waited for the woman to finish packing so that they could go to dinner. He knew better than to try to pack his suitcase when she hadn't finished packing hers yet. There would be no room on the bed. The woman had been upstairs preparing for their vacation for four hours, and he was getting hungry. He couldn't imagine what was taking so long. He sighed deeply, and climbed the stairs to see how she was doing. He gazed at clothing laid out on every conceivable space and on every door in both bedrooms and bathrooms.

He approached the woman with startled eyes, and asked with disbelief, "*Are you moving out?*"

Too Much of Everything – The Husband and Wife's Story

High Life Is Demanding – Never before in her life had the wife pined more for a simpler life. She had lived the high life of private jet travel, designer clothes, fine wines, fancy cars, and expensive jewelry. She didn't want to keep up with all those things in that lifestyle, and she felt tired of trying.

Sensible Choices – Recently, the husband and the wife decided to keep their old cars, and take them for regular servicing instead of buying new cars. The couple gave up designer water, and let the water cooler go back to the dealer. The wife walked away from the hairdresser, let her blonde hair grow out to shiny white, and stopped getting haircuts more than once a year. The husband and wife stopped buying expensive clothes, and now purchased durable and sensible clothing only when needed. They ended extravagant gift buying at Christmas. They used their reward miles for traveling, both air and hotel, and searched for good deals wherever possible. They gave up the gardener, and the wife did the work herself for an hour each morning.

Too Many Events – The husband and the wife gave up their annual Jazz Jubilee event for all their family and friends at Mammoth Mountain. *We did it for twenty years, but now we're moving on to new horizons*, thought the wife. They ended their subscriptions for the opera, the Ahmanson Theater, the box at the Hollywood Bowl, and the Greek Theater. Instead, the couple attended the free concerts around their neighborhood, and limited their theater events to a few at the local regional theater. *Now, we have time to go out to dinner with friends!* The husband speculated.

Fewer Foods for Gatherings – When the husband and the wife planned family gatherings, the wife cooked no more than two things, and made a simple salad. At the last luncheon they had, the wife made toastettes with cream cheese and bruschetta. The husband grilled the Cajun-coated lamb chops, and the wife made a strawberry salad. In the past, she would have made everything from the appetizer to the pies. Nowadays, the couple would rather enjoy their friends and family, and actually have a chance to visit with them than to have their time overwhelmed with cooking and serving.

Simpler Ways to Vacation – When the husband and the wife traveled, they tried to keep the extracurricular activities to a minimum, and skipped the fancy meals. Simple foods usually satisfied them just as much. Often, the husband and the wife shared a meal so that they didn't eat too much. They walked instead of taking a taxi if they wanted to go to a restaurant. They bought the seven-up for the wife's wine spritzers at the grocery store, and took it with them when they went out to eat.

Prohibited Garage Sales – A lot of stuff lied around the husband and the wife's house that was a result of the high life, more things than they could possibly use in their lifetime. The wife owned a preponderance of a particular designer, which currently sold at inflated prices on E-Bay, and fetched a fair amount at garage sales. However, the couple lived in a housing complex, which prohibited them from having a garage sale.

A Family in Despair – A family needed money to pay rent on their apartment, and was in despair. The son lost his job, and the mom cleaned four houses a week, not enough to support them. The husband and the wife knew what they had to do. They started in one corner of their home, and worked their way through every inch of space, drawer, and closet. They employed self-discipline through the process. They set aside *every* single item that they had not used or worn in a year. When they finished the process, the merchandise, including diamonds and high-priced clothing, filled an entire bedroom almost to the ceiling. It was inconceivable to them how many unnecessary things they had accumulated.

Faith and Good Works – The husband and the wife knew that faith and good works were a lot like good nutrition: the result is evident in a person's appearance just as good works are apparent from a person's faith. They gave everything to the family who couldn't pay their rent. The family sold the designer clothing on E-Bay, and had a huge garage sale. They earned enough money to pay their rent for six months and sustain them until the son could find another job.

Relief with a Simpler Life – Recently, for the first time, the wife sat in church wearing jeans instead of designer clothing. She felt wonderful to have a simpler life. The couple felt relieved to rid themselves of the burden of maintaining the high life, and it felt *great* to put faith into action.

Usefulness Expires – When the wife packs for vacation now, she is done within thirty minutes. If you have a multitude of things that you don't need or use, pass them on to someone else before their usefulness expires. Getting rid of the clutter is mind liberating.

Inspiration and Motivation

Anecdote

The woman hurriedly finished washing the dishes, gave the dogs their medicines, changed the laundry, and then grabbed her gardening apron and ran outside. She worked furiously with the loppers cutting down the branches that threatened to topple her trellis.

"This wall of growth needs a haircut, chop, chop!" she remarked as she chuckled to herself.

The man heard the woman breaking off large branches, and then hauling the wheelbarrow, loudly down the long sidewalk in the side yard, clunkety-clunking all the way. He emerged from his office with concern that she was going to overdo it.

"Is there something I can do to help?" He asked her.

"Yes, saw off all that pyracantha sticking up above the fence while I haul all these clippings out to the street before the garbage truck comes," she clipped with authority. The man obediently retrieved the saw, and went to work.

In the meantime, the woman buzzed around the yard sweeping up the mess that she had made. She dumped the clippings, returned her pail and the wheelbarrow to their designated locations, and jogged to the back yard.

"I'm going to exercise before it gets too late," she told the man in clipped staccato.

"Okay honey," the man replied and shook his head back and forth.

Every morning it was the same thing. She accomplished as much as she could in the yard within an hour, and bee-lined it to the recumbent bike where she would ride on the hill program for one hour. After that, she did pushups and sit-ups, and then stretches. The whole routine took two and a half hours every morning. She took Sundays off to replenish her body, go to church, and out to lunch. Before she cleaned up and returned downstairs to make lunch each day, she caught a few rays in her bikini in the sun on the front porch, a welcome respite after her morning of whirlwind activities. She had been doing the same thing for decades, and he wondered if she would ever tire of it.

The man finished sawing off the pyracantha, returned the saw to the garage, and climbed the stairs to talk to the woman. The woman watched television while her legs spun the pedals at high speed.

The main smiled at her and said, "I'm going for a walk around the lake." He started to leave, but then turned and inquired of her, "Don't you ever get tired of working out so much?"

"You know what they taught me at school, vigorous exercise at least five days a week for more than a half hour reduces my risk for breast or endometrial cancer by sixty-five percent! Now that I'm sixty years old, I don't do it just for shape and weight control. I do it to ward off cancer. It's even more important that it used to be!" She exclaimed with irritation that he would question her motivation.

"Okay then, *I am out of here!*" He cried back at her with the same vigor, and trotted off for his four-mile walk around the lake.

Inspire Others

You are the underdog of inspiration for those around you. Take your greatest weakness and change it to make it your boldest strength. When you do that, then the other weaknesses will follow into success.

Empower yourself with health and happiness, to fill yourself with strength and joy. Who you are now does not define who you can become. Keep growing towards the person whom you want to be. Start with one thing, and conquer that problem. You'll feel nothing but better. Begin to mold yourself into the ideal person you'd like to be, and enjoy the second half of your life more than any other time that you have lived!

Who you are *never* limits your ability to improve. Sum up your shortcomings and do something about it! The only thing that limits you is doubt in yourself. Get over it, and become a believer in yourself. Change your worst weakness into your greatest strength. If you think you can't do it, remember these people:

Moses stuttered.

Franklin Delano Roosevelt ruled the country from a wheelchair.

Helen Keller was deaf and blind.

John F. Kennedy had asthma.

Abraham Lincoln suffered from melancholia.

Vincent Van Gogh had epilepsy.

Charles Darwin had an obsessive-compulsive disorder.

Thomas Edison was deaf.

Zane Grey, the prolific writer, was an unsuccessful dentist.

Whistler, the painter, flunked out of West Point.

Shakespeare only learned a small amount of reading and writing in school.

Mozart wrapped his hands in socks to stay warm enough to write his immortal music.

Augustus Toplady wrote the hymn, "Rock of Ages," on a playing card in a rainstorm while under the shelter of a large rock.

George Washington was dyslexic.

Nelson Rockefeller had learning disabilities.

Winston Churchill had attention deficit disorder, and was bipolar.

Harry Truman had extreme vision problems.

Verdi composed *Ave Maria* at the age of eighty-five.

Grandma Moses took up painting at the age of seventy-seven.

Michelangelo worked on his sculptures until he died at the age of eighty-nine.

Arthur Fiedler conducted the Boston Pops into his eighties.

Will and Ariel Durant wrote the massive ten-volume *History of Civilization* between the ages of sixty-nine and eighty-nine.

You are the underdog of inspiration for those around you. Your dreams can become realities through persistence. Get motivated. Jonathan Swift, the author of *Gulliver's Travels*, once said, "Although men are accused of not knowing their own weakness, yet perhaps few know their own strength. It is in men as in soils, where sometimes there is a vein of gold which the owner knows not of."

This time of your life is a defining moment that can change you. Lead the way to a new reality.

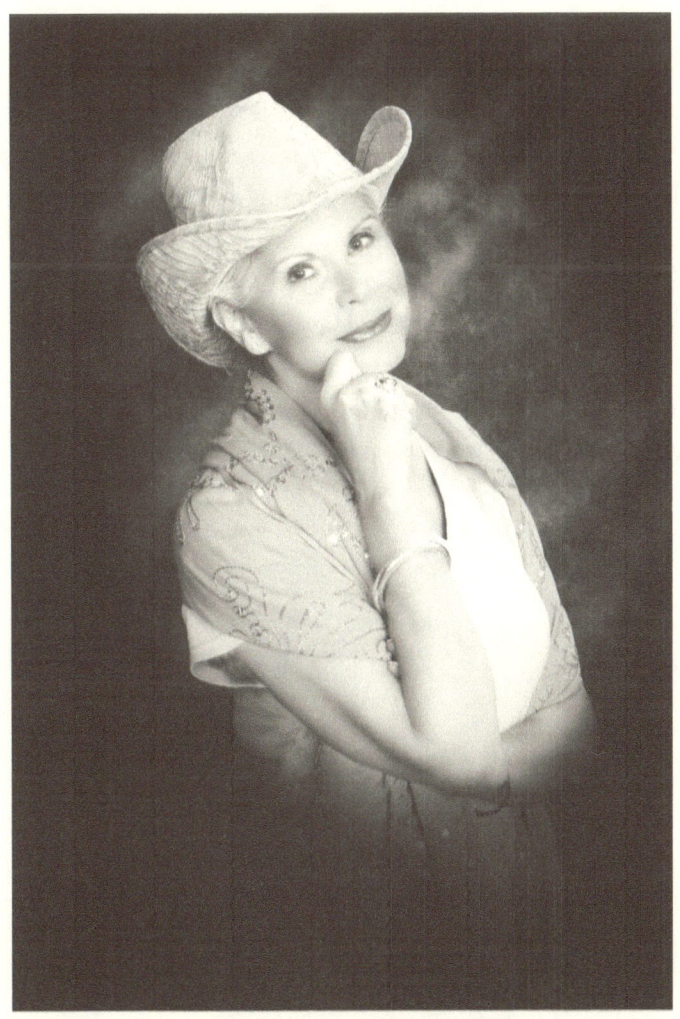

Photo by Lukas VanDyke

About the Author

Peggy grew up on a large dairy farm in Farmington, Minnesota. As a young woman, she rode the countryside on her magnificent American Saddlebred horse, Blaze King. Peggy Lee is a singer, pianist, composer, arranger, lyricist, equestrian, physical fitness fanatic, and fiction and non-fiction writer.

Peggy formerly owned and operated a nationwide consulting company for the financial industry. She has written hundreds of scholastic, business, and motivational books for colleges and corporations. Currently, Peggy is working on three series of faith-based fiction novels, and one series of non-fiction books.

Peggy met Don on a beach in Hawaii thirty years ago. They have been back to visit over fifty times. Currently, they live in Calabasas, California with their two little West Highland White Terriers: Daisy Lou and MacGregor.

The Faith Fiction Series
Innocence: Simplicity of Spirit
Confidence: Reliance on the Spirit
Consequence: Importance of the Spirit
Common Sense: Listening to the Spirit
Providence: Leading of the Spirit – Coming Soon

The Spirit Series
The Spirit Moves
The Spirit Guides: Insights from Everyday Life
The Spirit Praises: A Perfect Little Gift Book from Heaven
Available on www.Barnes&Noble.com and www.Amazon.com
and www.Borders.com

Peggy's Contact Information
www.sexyatsixty.us.com
http://sexyatsixtylivewell.blogspot.com
sexyatsixty@live.com

www.ingramcontent.com/pod-product-compliance
Lightning Source LLC
Chambersburg PA
CBHW020511290526
45786CB00002B/553